ACTIVATED CHARCOAL

Antidote, Remedy, and Health Aid

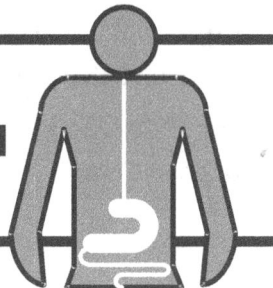

by

David O. Cooney, Ph.D.

I0038979

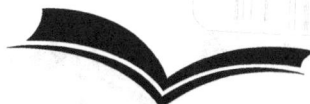

TEACH Services, Inc.
P U B L I S H I N G
www.TEACHServices.com • (800) 367-1844

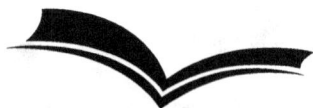

Copyright © 2016 TEACH Services, Inc.

Copyright © 1988 David O. Cooney

ISBN-13: 978-1-4796-0335-0 (Paperback)

ISBN-13: 978-1-4796-0336-7 (ePub)

ISBN-13: 978-1-4796-0337-4 (Mobi)

Library of Congress Control Number: 95-61283

Published by

TEACH Services, Inc.
P U B L I S H I N G
www.TEACHServices.com ● (800) 367-1844

Table of Contents

Chapter 7

Preface

Activated charcoal, long known to the ancients as a substance of therapeutic value in a variety of maladies, has recently been "rediscovered" to be of great general use as an oral antidote for drug overdoses and poisonings. Within the last 15 years, orally administered activated charcoal has been proven to be highly effective in reducing the systemic absorption (i.e., transfer from the gastrointestinal tract into the rest of the body) of analgesics and antipyretics, sedatives and hypnotics, alkaloids, tricyclic antidepressants, cardiac glycosides, solvents, and a wide variety of other kinds of drugs and chemicals. The effectiveness of activated charcoal in binding drugs and poisons within the gastrointestinal tract (therefore preventing their transfer into the rest of the body) has been demonstrated emphatically by a host of studies in humans, dogs, rabbits, pigs, sheep, rats, and other animals.

Oral activated charcoal has also recently been recognized as an aid for treating gastrointestinal disturbances. And, poultices made of charcoal pastes have been found to be effective for treating skin wounds, itching, and insect bites and stings.

It is rather surprising that prior to about 15 years ago, activated charcoal was essentially neglected, considering that its therapeutic effects had already been extensively reported in the medical literature. This neglect perhaps resulted from the fact that medical personnel were never really aware of how and why activated charcoal really works. Such a lack of knowledge would explain the origin of the absurd notion, prevalent in the 1950s, that burnt toast be used in place of activated charcoal. "Universal antidote" is another example of a concoction which, on a chemical basis, can be shown to be decidedly inferior to plain activated charcoal as a general antidote. The promotion and acceptance of such ill-founded notions undoubtedly did considerable harm to the reputation of activated charcoal and deterred people from using it.

Fortunately, the virtues of activated charcoal have finally been recognized, if still not completely understood, by the medical community. Nevertheless, very few private homes today have activated charcoal on hand as a ready antidote, remedy, and health-aid. And so there continues to be a wide gap between the appreciation of charcoal by medical researchers and the acceptance and utilization of charcoal by the general public.

This publication represents an attempt to gather together most of what has been reported to date on the use of activated charcoal as an oral antidote and as a remedy for other ailments. In addition to reviewing much recent research on the antidotal use of charcoal for a wide variety of drugs and poisons, we review what was known about charcoal by our ancestors, beginning at about 1500 B.C. A wide range of adsorption studies involving activated charcoal and viruses, bacteria, bacterial toxins, fungal toxins, etc., are also reviewed. These studies may form the basis for future expansion of the use of charcoal for medical purposes.

David O. Cooney

Chapter 1
Introduction

Acute incidents involving the accidental or intentional ingestion of drugs, poisons, and various household chemicals continue
to be a serious problem. In the United States, on the order of
150,000 incidents of this sort are annually reported to poison control centers. Hayden and Comstock (1975) have estimated that
about 365,000 admissions per year to intensive care units in U.S.
hospitals are due to drug overdoses or poisonings.

Two initial approaches to the emergency treatment of such
cases have been frequently used: induced vomiting with syrup of
ipecac or gastric lavage (repeated washing and pumping of the
stomach using essentially water). A number of studies have shown
that induced vomiting is more efficient, less time-consuming,
and less traumatic than lavage. Because syrup of ipecac is relatively safe and can be administered easily in the home, many people have recommended it highly. However, ipecac is not always
safe—it has been implicated in cardiac toxicity when it was used to
induce vomiting in patients overdosed with phenothiazines.

Ipecac syrup also takes considerable time to work. In one study (Robertson, 1962) it was found that of 250 patients given 20ml ipecac syrup, the average delay before vomiting was 19 minutes. Although this may seem to be a long time, even more time is probably needed to carry out a stomach lavage. for quickly absorbed drugs like barbiturates, neither induced vomiting nor stomach lavage may be rapid enough. Another factor against ipecac is that it is ineffective against drugs which inhibit the regurgitation response (e.g., chlorpromazine).

Other induced vomiting agents that have been recommended in the past are now considered to be dangerous. For example, several deaths have occurred with table salt solutions. Other agents, like copper sulfate and potassium antimony tartrate, are relatively toxic; therefore, if vomiting fails to occur, poisoning from such agents will follow.

When the patient is unconscious or very lethargic, induced vomiting cannot be employed, and gastric lavage is often used. However, because some of the drug or poison is hidden in the recesses of the stomach and is thus not accessible to the lavage tube, lavage is often not very efficient. The efficiencies of both induced vomiting and stomach lavage have been reported to be on the order of 40% or less. One careful study (Corby et al., 1968) has shown, for example, an average recovery of stomach contents of only 27% (range 0–77%) from ipecac-induced vomiting.

Oral dilution with large volumes of water has also been recommended as a first aid treatment for overdoses. It was believed that such dilution would retard the rate of absorption of the toxic material from the stomach or intestines into the body as a whole. However, Henderson, Picchioni, and Chin (1966) have clearly shown that oral dilution often greatly increases the rate of absorption into the body as a whole, the reason for this being that dilution promotes emptying from the stomach, which exposes the drug or poison to the larger absorptive surfaces of the intestines. This fact also suggests that stomach lavage might similarly induce more rapid absorption, at least for a while.

In summary, it appears that the time delay required to promote induced vomiting or to carry out lavage, combined with the unpredictable and low efficiencies of these two methods, makes them unsatisfactory in many cases.

A better approach, which has been rediscovered in recent years, involves the use of activated charcoal. Activated charcoal has the ability to adsorb a wide variety of drugs or poisons. It is nontoxic, does not lose its potency if kept in a closed container, and can be conveniently administered in the home. Studies have shown that slurries of powdered activated charcoal in water are well accepted by both adults and children.

Activated charcoal has been proven effective in tests with all kinds of subjects (humans, dogs, rats, rabbits, sheep, pigs) for many different types of overdoses. The charcoal adsorbs most drugs and poisons fast and in significant amounts.

Charcoal is a poor adsorbent only for simple acids, alkalis, and salts (e.g., NaCl, $FeSO_4$, etc.). Some of the chemical compounds effectively adsorbed by activated charcoal are listed in Table 1.

Charcoal adsorbs most drugs and poisons fast and in significant amounts.

TABLE 1
Some Substances Effectively Adsorbed by Activated Charcoal

BARBITURATES		
Amobarbital	Cyclobarbital	Phenobarbital
Aprobarbital	Hexobarbital	Quinalbital
Barbital	Pentobarbital	Secobarbital
NON BARBITURATE HYPNOTICS, SEDATIVES AND TRANQUILIZERS		
Ethchlorvynol	Prochlorperazine	Diphenoxylate Hydrochloride
Glutethimide	Fluphenazine	2, 4 Dichlorophe-noxyacetic Acid
Diphenylhydantoin	Thioridazine	Morphine
Diazepam	Chlorpheniramine	Opium
Chlorpromazine	Propanolamine	Meprobamate
Promazine	Phenylpropanol-amine	
Promethazine	Tripelennamine	
ANTIDEPRESSANTS		
Amphetamine	Imipramine	Desipramine
Nortriptyline		
ALCOHOLS		
Ethanol	Benzyl Alcohol	Isopropyl Alcohol
Ethylene Glycol		
ANALGESICS		
Acetylsalicylic Acid (Aspirin)	Methyl Salicylate	Opium
Salicylic Acid	Acetaminophen	Pentazocine
Salicylimide	Mefenamic Acid	Propoxyphene
Sodium Salicylate	Mefenamic Acid	

ANTIMICROBIALS/ANTI-CANCER AGENTS		
Penicillin	Quinacrine	Primaquine
Sulfanilamide	Quinine	Colchicine
Isoniazid	Quinidine	Chloroquine
METALS/INORGANICS		
Antimony	Lead	Silver
Arsenic	Mercuric Chloride	Tin
Calcium	Potassium	Titanium
Cyanides	Phosphorus	
Iodine	Phosphate	
PLANT/ANIMAL TOXINS/HERBICIDES/INSECTICIDES		
Aconite	Digitalis	Malathion
Amaniti Phalloidin	Elaterin	Paralytic Shellfish Toxin
Atropine Sulfate	Hemlock	Quinine
Cantharides	Ipecac	Stramonium
Cocaine	Muscarine	Strychnine
Chlordane	Nicotine	Veratrum
Delphinium	Opium	Yohimbine
DDT	Parathion	
SOLVENTS		
Kerosene	Camphor	Phenol
CARDIOVASCULAR AGENTS		
Digitalis	ß -Methyldigoxin	Ergotamine
Digoxin	Quinine	Propantheline
Digitoxin	Quinidine	
ENDOGENOUS TOXINS		
Bilirubin	Creatinine	Uric Acid

(continued on next page)

MISCELLANEOUS		
Camphor	Potassium	Doxycycline
Oxalates	Permanganate	Diphenylhydantoin
Methylene Blue	N-Methyl	Sulfonamides
Phenolphthalein	Carbamate	Cimetidine
Phenprocoumon	Chlorpheniramine	
Hexachlorophene	Theophylline	

The consensus now emerging among clinical physicians is that the best way of handling overdoses consists of the administration of large amounts (100g or more) of powdered charcoal as a slurry in water. This procedure should be carried out in the home (if possible) or in the emergency room. If the patient is not conscious, the activated charcoal slurry can be administered in the emergency room by the use of a stomach tube. Ipecac could also be used, but is less effective, and since charcoal effectively adsorbs the active constituents of ipecac (Cooney, 1978), the syrup of ipecac should not be given before the charcoal.

An impressive testimonial to the benefits of activated charcoal has been stated by Hayden and Comstock (1975). They recount their own clinical experience with treating poisoned and over-dosed patients in intensive care wards. From 500 patients not treated with charcoal and 1000 who were, Hayden and Comstock found that administering activated charcoal after gastric lavage effectively reduced further drug absorption, as indicated by a leveling off of central nervous system (CNS) depression within about 2 hours. When charcoal was not used, progressive CNS depression occurred for up to 48 hours or longer. They estimate that the use of charcoal could reduce the average stay in an intensive care unit of 3 or 4 days by at least 1 day. This alone could save over 70 million dollars in the value of care avoided, not to mention the great benefits of reductions in morbidity and mortality which can also be expected.

Chapter 2
Historical Background

I.   TERMINOLOGY

The terms "activated charcoal," "activated carbon," and "active carbon," all occur in the literature and are generally used interchangeably.

Although some scientists prefer the adjective "active" to "activated," almost all charcoals in modern practical use have been purposely "activated" by taking the charcoal resulting from the controlled charring of the starting material and subjecting it to an oxidizing gas such as

The terms "activated charcoal," "activated carbon," and "active carbon," all occur in the literature and are generally used interchangeably.

steam or air at elevated temperatures. (This enhances the adsorptive power of the charcoal by developing an extensive internal network of fine pores in the material.) Thus, the adjective "activated" is most appropriate and will be employed hereafter. Concerning the second half of the term, engineers and most manufacturers seem to prefer the term "carbon," whereas the *U.S. Pharmacopoeia*, most of the medical community, and a few manufacturers prefer "charcoal." Regardless of the starting material used, no charcoal is purely carbon, but is rather a combination of carbon plus a few other elements. Thus, the term "carbon" is not strictly correct. For this reason, and because of its overwhelming traditional usage in the medical literature, we shall use the term "activated charcoal" throughout this work. It should be mentioned that prior to about 1900, charcoals were not activated (the activation process had not been invented). Hence, the proper term for such materials is simply "charcoal."

II. EARLY HISTORY

The use of charcoal for medicinal purposes is ancient. In an Egyptian papyrus of 1550 B.C., various kinds of charcoal are specified for medicinal use. Over succeeding centuries, those who practiced as physicians believed greatly in the healing properties and therapeutic values of wood charcoal. In the times of Hippocrates (400 B.C.) and Pliny (50 A.D.), wood charcoal was used to treat epilepsy, vertigo, chlorosis, and anthrax. These practices gradually fell into disuse, but were still mentioned, often even into the nineteenth century. D. M. Kehls (1793) wrote of the external application of charcoal to gangrenous ulcers to remove bad odors. Charcoal was also recommended for internal use in the treatment of "fievre putride" at a dosage of 1/16 oz. charcoal six times daily. Kehls also recommended that charcoal suspended in water be used as a mouthwash, and, additionally, at the first indications of any bilious condition (build-up of excess bile).

The discovery of how charcoal really works, that is, of the phenomenon of adsorption as we presently understand it, is generally attributed to Scheele (Dietz, 1944), who in 1773 described some experiments on gases exposed to charcoal. The charcoal was found to adsorb many types of gases to a significant extent. In the area of liquid phase systems, the earliest notice of adsorption seems to have been in 1785, when Lowitz observed that charcoal would decolorize many liquids. Soon after, wood charcoal was used to clarify cane sugar in a sugar refinery.

During the nineteenth century many attempts were made to produce decolorizing charcoals from other sources. In 1822, Bussy found that by heating blood with potash, an effective charcoal was produced. Hunter, in 1865, reported on the great capacity of a charcoal derived from coconut shells for adsorbing gases. Other charcoals were made by Lee, in 1863, from peat, and by Winser and Swindells, in 1868, from paper mill wastes (Hassler, 1963).

The charcoals made in the 1800s, and before, were not activated in the sense we are familiar with. That is, they were made by charring alone, without any subsequent treatment using oxidizing gases. Thus, their adsorption abilities, while decent, were still far lower than that of modern activated charcoals. Ostrejko, a Russian, is credited with introducing the concept of activation. In 1900 and 1901 he patented several processes involving the treatment of charred matter with super-heated steam or carbon dioxide and showed that these greatly enhanced the adsorbing powers of the charcoals.

Gradually, over the period from 1870 to about 1920, more and more processes and source materials were tried. A complete list of source materials that have been tried would include such diverse materials as blood, cereals, fish, fruit pits, kelp, corncobs, rice hulls, and distillery waste. However, the superiority of charcoals made from certain sources, and the costs of purchasing and processing different materials, have by now reduced the number of practical choices. Today, charcoals are essentially made only from petroleum coke, coals (bituminous, lignite), peat, sawdust and wood char, paper mill waste (lignin), bone char, and coconut shells.

According to Holt and Holz (1963), the first systematic studies of charcoal as an antidote were performed in France in the early 1800s. A chemist named Bertrand studied arsenic poisoning in animals around 1811 and observed that charcoal was effective in preventing toxicity. It is claimed that in 1813 he gave a public demonstration of its effectiveness by swallowing 5g arsenic trioxide mixed with charcoal. Touery, a French pharmacist, also did studies using animals in the years 1820–1840, and in 1831 was reported to have swallowed a mixture of 15g charcoal and strychnine (in the amount of 10 times a lethal dose) as a demonstration for the French Academy of Medicine. According to Andersen (1946), an American physician named Hort succeeded, in 1834, in saving a patient from bichloride of mercury poisoning by having the patient consume large amounts of powdered charcoal.

Garrod (1846) reported some extensive early studies he performed in England using strychnine and other poisons administered to dogs, cats, rabbits, and guinea pigs. He carefully studied the effectiveness of charcoal as affected by (1) the poison dose, (2) the charcoal dose, and (3) the time interval between the ingestion of the poison and the charcoal. Garrod found charcoal to be effective, not only against strychnine, but also against opium, morphine, aconite, ipecac, veratrum, elaterium, stramonium, cantharides, delphinium, hemlock, and mineral poisons, such as bichloride of mercury, silver nitrate, and lead salts.

Rand (1848), an American physician, extended Garrod's type of studies to humans. in a paper published in 1848, he reported on observations made using various drugs, including digitalis, morphine, strychnine, arsenic, camphor, iodine, and bichloride of mercury. He, like Garrod, determined what ratio of charcoal to drug was required to reduce clinical symptoms of toxicity to a barely detectable level.

Kunzova (1937) reported some interesting studies with frogs. Strychnine was dissolved in a dilute salt solution, treated with various charcoals, filtered, and then injected into the lymph sacs of frogs. When the ratio of charcoal to strychnine was 65:1, convulsions appeared in 25 minutes; when the ratio was larger, convulsions failed to appear. Little variations between the different charcoals were observed. It appeared that the amount of charcoal needed to adsorb 1mg strychnine ranged only between 65 and 76mg. Some similar studies were reported by Saunders et al.

(1931). They shook activated charcoal with solutions of various drugs, filtered them, and injected the filtrates into dogs. Strychnine, brucine, adrenalin, histamine, and tyramine were completely inactivated. Acetylcholine and ephedrine solutions were partly inactivated.

During the late 1800s and early 1900s there continued to be many reports on the efficacy of charcoal as an antidote, mainly in the European literature. In America, interest grew in charcoal as an aid in curing intestinal disorders. For example, the 1908 catalog of Sears, Roebuck and Co. (reprinted in 1969) carried the following advertisement:

WILLOW CHARCOAL TABLETS
Every person is well acquainted with the great benefit derived from willow charcoal in gastric and intestinal disorder, indigestion, dyspepsia, heartburn, sour or acid stomach, gas upon the stomach, constant belching, fetid breath, all gaseous complications and for the removal of the offensive odor from the breath after smoking.

A similar advertisement of the same period touts claims of anti-bacterial and anti-parasitic activity:

BRAGG'S VEGETABLE CHARCOAL AND CHARCOAL BISCUITS
Absorb all impurities in the stomach and bowels. Give a healthy tone to the whole system, effectually warding off cholera, smallpox, typhoid, and all malignant fevers. Invaluable for indigestion, flatulence, etc. Eradicate worms in children. Sweeten the breath.

It was not until much later that scientific research demonstrated that most of the claims made in such advertisements are indeed valid. It is now known that activated charcoal can adsorb poisons, bacterial toxins, and such, in the gastrointestinal tract.

Chapter 3
Fundamentals of Activated Charcoal and the Adsorption Process

I. THE MANUFACTURE OF ACTIVATED CHARCOAL

Although those persons who use activated charcoal for medical or remedial purposes may not require detailed information on how activated charcoals are manufactured, a general knowledge of such can be useful in understanding how different adsorption properties arise. This will help one develop a feeling for why various activated charcoals often behave differently as antidotes, and may permit one to more rationally select the best charcoal for a given application.

While most carbonaceous substances can be converted into activated charcoal, the final properties of the charcoal will nevertheless reflect to a considerable extent the nature of the source material. This is particularly true with respect to the hardness of the final product, e.g., coconut shells yield a strong, dense charcoal which resists mechanical abrasion well.

A great many methods of manufacture of activated charcoals exist, and indeed hundreds of patents have been issued covering specific procedures. However, most processes can be said to consist of the charring (or pyrolysis or carbonization) of the starting material, followed usually (but not always) by a stage of controlled oxidation. This latter stage is what is meant by "activation" of the charcoal.

A. CARBONIZATION (CHARRING)

This step is usually carried out by heating the source material to temperatures ranging between 600 and 900°C in the absence of air. Sometimes limited amounts of air are allowed and the source material undergoes a slow burning process. Development of a porous material during this first step has been found to be aided greatly by incorporating metallic chlorides in the starting mixture. A typical example of this is the European process in which a concentrated zinc chloride solution is mixed with pulverized peat or sawdust, dried, and carbonized in in a kiln at 600–700°C. The zinc salt is removed from the product by washing it with dilute acid and water. If only large pores are desired in the charcoal (as in those used for decolorizing sugars, where the color molecules to be adsorbed are fairly large and which, therefore, can penetrate only large pores) then this first step may be all that is needed. However, most charcoals are subjected to a second step called oxidation.

B. ACTIVATION WITH OXIDIZING GASES

The basic character of a charcoal is determined in the first (pyrolysis) step, and the subsequent oxidation step must be tailored to fit in with the first stage. Oxidation is usually carried out using steam, although air (and more rarely, CO_2) is sometimes employed. Temperatures are normally in the range of 600–900°C. Under the proper conditions, the oxidizing gas selectively erodes the internal surfaces of the charcoal, develops a greater and finer network of pores in the charcoal, and converts the atoms lying along the surfaces to specific chemical forms (e.g., oxides) which may have selective powers of adsorption.

The various changes which occur do not all happen at the same rate. Some types of changes develop early and some develop late in the process. Depending on the properties desired, the total time allowed for activation is a very important variable. Thus, the ability of a charcoal to adsorb different materials can depend strongly on the activation time. The primary effect of time is on the sizes of the pores which develop. As time goes on, a succeedingly larger number of pores are generated and the internal surface area gradually increases. However, as the process continues, solid material separating adjacent pores may be eaten away; the net result is the generation of larger pores and a reduction in the total internal surface area.

II. THE PROPERTIES OF ACTIVATED CHARCOAL

A. COMPOSITION

Activated charcoals contain constituents derived from the source material or from ingredients (such as metallic chlorides) added during manufacture. Typical compositions of activated charcoals are shown in Table 2.

TABLE 2:
Elemental Composition of Activated Charcoals*

Charcoal	Ash	Carbon	Hydrogen	Sulfur	Nitrogen
1	4.3	94.4	1.1	0.04	0.62
2	3.2	91.7	1.7	0.07	0.38
3	1.2	95.3	0.6	0.62	0.54
4	2.0	87.5	2.2	0.16	0.39

*All values in percent by weight. Adapted from Hassler (1963)

The "ash" consists of the residue remaining when a sample of the charcoal, placed in a porcelain crucible, is heated in air in a furnace at 600°C until the carbon has been entirely burned. Ashes range typically from about 1 to 5% of the original charcoal weight. It is common also to designate the amount of ash which is water soluble and the amount of ash which is acid soluble. As Table 3 shows, the acid–soluble part is on the order of 1% or less of the original charcoal weight and the water-soluble portion is about 1.3% or less. Some of the constituents of the ash that are commonly found are iron, calcium, sodium, copper, sulfates, chlorides, and phosphates.

The 19th edition of the *U.S. Pharmacopoeia* (USP), published in 1975, specifically states that USP activated charcoals should be fine, black, odorless, and tasteless powders which are free from gritty matter and which possess the following additional characteristics: less than 15% weight loss on drying, less than 4% residue after ignition (i.e., ash), less than 3.5% acid-soluble substances, less than 0.2% alcohol soluble substances, less than 0.15% sulfate, less than 0.02% chloride, and less than 0.005% heavy metals content. To meet these standards, USP-grade activated charcoals are normally washed with acid to remove the major part of the inorganic constituents. Any components of the ash not extracted by acid washing would not normally be solubilized when the charcoal is subsequently used.

B. PORE VOLUME AND PORE SIZE DISTRIBUTION

Pore volume represents the total volume of the pores in a charcoal particle per unit weight of the charcoal. Values are usually on the order of 0.7–1.5 ml/g.

Activated charcoals contain a complex network of pores of various shapes and sizes. The shapes are irregular, branched,

Activated charcoals contain a complex network of pores of various shapes and sizes.

and interconnected by passages which may or may not be constricting. Pore sizes range from less than 0.1 millionths of a centimeter to more than one hundredth of a centimeter. The so-called pore size distribution depends on the source materials used and on the method and extent of activation. Pores are often classified as macropores, micropores, and transitional pores. Through well-established methods, which we shall not review here, it is possible to determine the relative numbers of pores of a given size. Table 3 shows typical pore-size distribution data.

Table 3:
Some Properties of Powdered Charcoals

Property	Darco G-60	Darco S-51	Darco KB	Norit A	Norit SG Extra
Source material	Lignite	Lignite	Wood	Peat	Peat
Surface area (m²/g)	600	650	1450	720	810
Bulk Density (g/ml)	0.4	0.51	0.45	0.34	0.30
Pore Volume (ml/g)	1.0	1.0	1.5	—	—
Ash (%)	3.5	—	—	5.9	6.0
Acid Solubles (%)	1.0	—	—	—	0.5
H_2O Solubles (%)	0.3	1.0	1.3	0.3	0.2
Moisture (%)	8	8	25	10	10
Particle size (%)					
< 100 mesh	95	98	99	98-100	98-100
< 325 mesh	70	70	70	60-65	60-55
Pore volume distribution (%)					
< 20 Å	10	15	27	—	—
< 20-50 Å	10	15	27	—	—
< 50-100 Å	30	10	13	—	—

Property	Darco G-60	Darco S-51	Darco KB	Norit A	Norit SG Extra
< 100-500 Å	35	20	30	—	—
> 500 Å	15	30	10	—	—
Mean Pore radius (Å)	25	30	23	—	—
Å = Angstroms (an Angstrom is 0.00000001 centimeter.) Mesh = Particle size expressed in terms of the mesh size of a screen that it will just barely pass through (e.g., a 100-mesh has 100 wires per inch horizontally and vertically.)					

Pore size distributions are useful in selecting charcoals with high adsorptive capacities for particular types of molecules. For removal of "color bodies" from liquids, a charcoal having fairly large pores is needed, since color bodies are of relatively high molecular weight. For gas adsorption, small pores are best. For adsorption of drugs and poisons, which are of moderate molecular size, a charcoal having many pores of an intermediate size would be best.

C. SURFACE AREA

Internal surface areas are usually measured by a standard technique in which nitrogen gas is contacted with the activated charcoal at the atmospheric boiling point of liquid nitrogen (-196°C), at an initial pressure of less than 1 atm. The pressure is then raised slowly. As this occurs, nitrogen gradually condenses as a layer onto the internal surfaces. By measuring the amount of nitrogen required to form one complete layer, and knowing the area that a single N2 molecule covers, one can then compute the internal surface area of the charcoal sample used. Typical surface areas are in the range of 600–1500 M2/g, with 1000 M2/g being about average. Most of the internal surface area is associated with the smaller pores.

It should be pointed out in passing that even if a charcoal is very finely powdered, its external surface area will still be very small compared to the internal surface area. There have been misconceptions about this in the literature in which writers have implied that the great surface area of charcoal is due to its being finely divided. This implies that it is the external area which contributes most to the total surface area for adsorption. Such is not the case.

III. THE NATURE OF THE ADSORPTION PROCESS

The chemical nature of the internal surfaces created when charcoal is activated is such that the surface has an attraction for certain molecules if they are present in the liquid phase which fills the pores.

A.   THE LANGMUIR EQUATION

The Langmuir Equation is one of the more common expressions of the relation between the amount of a chemical species adsorbed and the concentration of the same chemical species in the liquid phase, at a given constant temperature.

The Langmuir Equation is given below, where Q is the amount of adsorbed chemical (in grams of chemical per gram of charcoal), C is the concentration of the chemical in the liquid (in grams of chemical per liter of solution), and K and Q_m are constants (i.e. specific numbers).

$$Q = \frac{KCQ_m}{1+KC}$$

The constants K and Q_m, which vary for each charcoal/chemical combination, can be determined from experimental data on Q versus C by straightforward methods. Q_m can be seen to be the value that Q levels out at as C gets large (i.e., it is the maximum adsorption capacity).

The shape of the Langmuir Equation for different K values is given below in Figure 1.

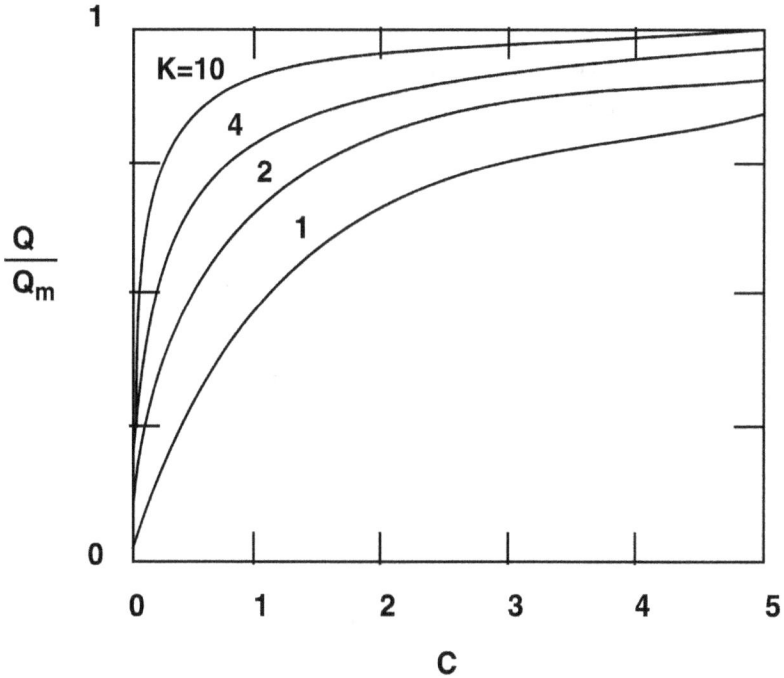

Figure 1. The Langmuir Equation for various K values

Note that the degree of adsorption of the chemical species rises sharply with the concentration of that species in the liquid, but tapers off at higher concentrations, as the available free surface for adsorption becomes more and more scarce.

B.   *NATURE OF THE ADSORBING SPECIES*

"Inorganic" compounds display a wide range of adsorbability. On one hand, salts like sodium chloride and potassium nitrate, which dissociate into positively charged and negatively charged portions when dissolved in water, are essentially not at all adsorbed by activated charcoal. On the other hand, non-dissociating species like iodine and mercuric chloride are very well adsorbed. The key factor seems to be whether the chemical exists in uncharged or in charged form in solution.

As for "organic" substances, which are of most interest to us, several generalizations can be made. The more "organic" the species is (i.e., of lower solubility in water), the better it is adsorbed. Also, an increase in size of such molecules usually enhances adsorption, especially for compounds that are similar. There is, in fact, a generalization known as Traube's rule which states: "the adsorption of organic substances from water solutions increases strongly and regularly as we ascend the homologous series." A homologous series is one such as CH_3OH, CH_3CH_2OH, $CH_3CH_2CH_2OH$, etc. The series consists of molecules that are very similar chemically, but which increase steadily in molecular weight as one ascends the series.

Chapter 4
Aspects of Antidotal Charcoal

At this point we shall digress from discussing the adsorption of specific drugs or poisons and will consider some of the more general aspects of antidotal charcoal. We will address the broad questions of what kind of charcoal to give, what physical form it should be in (e.g., tablets, powder), how much to give, and when it should be given. Other aspects of charcoal itself, namely, its toxicity and storage stability, will also be considered.

I.   SELECTION OF AN ACTIVATED CHARCOAL

There have been relatively few studies in which the adsorption abilities of different brands of activated charcoals have been compared. These studies show that, in general, charcoals having high internal surface areas tend to adsorb larger quantities of drugs and poisons than lower surface area charcoals, as one would expect.

The type of charcoal to select would be, in general, one that is relatively free of acid-leachable materials (i.e., an acid-washed charcoal), one that has a high internal surface area, and one whose pore-size distribution shows a predominance of pores that are intermediate in size. Nearly all "medicinal" type charcoals meet these criteria. Indeed, the requirements of the *U.S. Pharmacopoeia* essentially guarantee that a charcoal meet such standards.

It is *not* recommended that one attempt to prepare activated charcoal at home. The activation process requires very careful control of proper conditions. Additionally, acid-leaching to remove metals and other impurities is potentially hazardous and must be done according to exacting procedures.

II. CHARCOAL POWDER VERSUS TABLETED CHARCOAL

The great adsorption power of activated charcoal is primarily due to the very large internal surface areas associated with the numerous tiny pores which develop in the charcoal during activation.

The great adsorption power of activated charcoal is primarily due to the very large internal surface areas associated with the numerous tiny pores which develop in the charcoal during activation.

It is therefore clear that for charcoal to be effective in adsorbing drugs or poisons, one should maximize the ease of access of the drug or poison molecules to the internal surface. To adsorb, a drug or poison molecule must reach the external surface of the charcoal, diffuse inside, and then travel by molecular diffusion through the pore network until a vacant adsorption "site" is found. Molecular diffusion is an extremely slow process.

By dispersing a given weight of charcoal as fine particles (as opposed to larger granules), two advantages are gained: (1) a much larger external surface area is generated, and (2) the length of the diffusion paths inside the charcoal are reduced. The net effect is that, in general, the rate of uptake of the drug or poison by the charcoal will be inversely proportional to the particle size squared. Thus 325-mesh particles (0.043 mm diameter) compared to, for example, 20-mesh particles (0.833 mm diameter) will adsorb a drug $(0.833/0.043)^2$ or 375 times faster. In practice, if the fluid medium is not well agitated, the difference won't be quite this large, but will still be very appreciable. Thus, one should use powdered charcoal, indeed a finely powdered grade, for best results.

Tsuchiya and Levy (1972a) have compared the adsorption rates of a powdered charcoal and a commercially available (at this time, but perhaps no longer) tableted charcoal. The tablets, which weighed 0.44g each, contained 0.33g charcoal. The difference (0.11g) represents added ingredients required to produce the tablet form. Using phenylpropanolamine as a test drug, Tsuchiya and Levy found a very great difference in adsorption rates for the powder and tablet forms. Studies with human volunteers demonstrated that equal doses of charcoal powder and tablets reduced phenylpropanolamine absorption into the body as a whole by 73 and 48%, respectively. Actually, the tablets, though much less effective, were surprisingly adsorptive considering their long disintegration times. A second study with aspirin showed 38 and 15% reductions in absorption with the use of powdered and tableted charcoal, respectively. These studies make it very clear that any tableted or granular form of charcoal would be far less effective than finely powdered charcoal.

III. OPTIMUM DOSE AGE OF ACTIVATED CHARCOAL

The optimum dose of activated charcoal that should be given is a point of some contention. In an effort to determine what the

Tableted or granular form of charcoal would be far less effective than finely powdered charcoal.

optimum dose might be, Chin et al. (1973) did studies in which three drugs—sodium pentobarbital, chloroquine phosphate, and isoniazid—were given to rats, followed by charcoal in various amounts. The charcoal doses were one, two, four, or eight times the weight of drug employed. Table 4 shows representative tissue concentrations relative to animals that were not given any charcoal. What this study suggests is a rather obvious fact: the more charcoal, the better. The data do suggest that to be highly effective, an 8:1 ratio of charcoal to drug should be used. However, many investigations which have been carried out on fasted animals using a 5:1 ratio have shown charcoal to be quite effective.

TABLE 4:
Effect of Various Charcoal-to-Drug Ratios

	Percent Reduction in tissue concentration relative to controls (various ratios)			
Drug	**1:1**	**2:1**	**4:1**	**8:1**
Sodium pentobarbital	7.0	38.0	62.0	89.0
Chloroquine phosphate	20.0	30.0	70.0	96.0
Isoniazid	1.2	7.2	35.0	80.0

Adapted from Chin et al.(1973)

Other studies have, on the other hand, shown that too little charcoal is ineffective. For example, in a study by Levy and Tsuchiya (1969) it was shown that a charcoal-to-drug ratio of 1.9:1.0 had little effect on aspirin absorption in fasted human subjects. A ratio of 1.7:1.0 was totally ineffective in another study

(Chin, Picchioni, and Duplisse, 1970) in reducing glutethimide absorption in fasted dogs. It would thus appear that a 5:1 ratio is roughly a minimal figure. Many investigators, with this in mind, have recommended that a level twice as high (a 10:1 ratio) would be a safer rule-of-thumb.

The presence of food in the digestive tract is a factor that must also be taken into account. For example, Levy and Tsuchiya (1972) have shown that the percentage of a 1g aspirin dose absorbed into the body and subsequently recovered in the urine of human subjects, when 10g activated charcoal was given immediately after the aspirin, was 62.6% for fasted subjects and 75.9% for subjects who had eaten a standard breakfast 15 minutes before the test. Therefore, the action of the charcoal was inhibited by the presence of food. Atkinson and Azarnoff (1971), however, claim to have observed the opposite effect, i.e., much lower absorption of sodium salicylate into the body was found in tests with dogs when they had been fed I hour prior to the tests.

On one hand, it can be expected that food would reduce the effectiveness of charcoal because (1) it might prevent good contact of the drug and the charcoal (i.e., food might be a physical barrier separating the two), and (2) food decomposition products might compete with the drug for adsorption sites on the charcoal. On the other hand, the presence of food would undoubtedly slow down the rate of drug absorption into a person's system, thereby giving the charcoal more time in which to bind the drug. How these competing effects will balance may depend on the person, the type and amount of food eaten, the amounts of drug and charcoal ingested, the length of time between food and drug and charcoal ingestion, and the chemical characteristics of the drug (whether it is a quickly or slowly absorbed drug), and the effect of the drug on gastrointestinal contractions. The net result could easily be either an increased or decreased absorption into the body. Without definitive experiments, it is impossible to make any firmer statements on the net effect of the presence of food.

However, it should be noted that in an actual overdose or poisoning situation, the physician may have no knowledge of (1) the quantity of drug ingested, and (2) whether or not the digestive tract contains significant food. Additionally, it may not even be known what kind of drug was taken. Moreover, drugs vary enormously in their toxicities, rates of absorption, and the specific effects which overdoses produce (e.g., depression of respiration, convulsions, etc.). The physician is thus in a dilemma. The amount of charcoal cannot be computed using the 10:1 ratio concept if the weight of drug involved is unknown.

Therefore, several people have recommended certain fixed amounts. Dordoni et al. (1973) recommend 50g charcoal, as do Lawrence and McGrew (1975). Levy and Gwilt (1972) suggest a figure of 30–50g, and Levy and Houston (1976) recommend 50–100g. Comstock (1975) has suggested that no less than 100g be administered. Hayden and Comstock (1975), noting that textbooks that physicians use for reference often recommend a standard dose of 10g charcoal, stated that "in reality the dose of activated charcoal that should be administered to adsorb drugs from the gastrointestinal tract is in the range of 100 to 120g." Corby and Decker (1974) have pointed out, however, that since charcoal is harmless, the only limiting factor is the quantity the individual is willing to accept; accordingly, the optimum dose is the maximum that can be given practically. Nevertheless, it would seem that l00g charcoal would be sufficient for nearly all cases. For if a 10:1 ratio of charcoal to drug is really enough, then 100g charcoal would counteract 10g drug. This corresponds to one hundred 100mg barbiturate capsules, for example. (it is unlikely a typical overdose would involve much more than 10g of a drug.)

Repeated administration of activated charcoal after an adequate initial dose does not cause significant additional inhibition of drug/poison uptake into the body as a whole. Chin, Picchioni, and Duplisse (1969) have shown, for example, that repeated doses of activated charcoal in dogs at two 1-hour intervals after the administration of glutethimide or at two 12-hour intervals after administration of barbital were no more effective than a single dose of activated charcoal. However, for drugs that recycle back to the gastrointestinal system (by enterohepatic circulation, which involves the extraction of the drug from a person's blood stream by the liver and the subsequent excretion of the drug by the liver into the bile, with which it passes back to the intestinal tract when bile flows into the intestines), it may be possible to achieve lower tissue levels of the drug with additional doses of charcoal.

IV. EFFECT OF DELAY IN ADMINISTERING CHARCOAL

The effect of a delay in time between ingestion of a drug or poison and the administration of activated charcoal depends on the balance between two factors: (1) the duration of the time delay, and (2) the rate of absorption of the drug into the body as a whole. The latter process, in turn, will depend on how much food is in the digestive tract, the solubility of the drug or poison in gastrointestinal fluids, the effect of the drug or poison on the stomach emptying rate and on intestinal contractions, and the dosage form of the drug or poison (tablets, liquid, suspension, etc.).

In general, charcoal should be administered as soon as possible. Several investigators have suggested that a time of 30 minutes is a rough limit beyond which charcoal will be decidedly less effective. However, Levy and Tsuchiya (1972) have shown that when aspirin is administered from prolonged-release or delayed-release forms, charcoal is effective even if given several hours after the aspirin, as shown in Table 5.

In general, charcoal should be administered as soon as possible.

TABLE 5:
Effect of Delayed Administration

Subject	Time Delay (HR)	Dose recovered in the urine (%)	
		Tablets Alone	**With Charcoal**

A	3	90.5	38.0
B	3	85.5	68.8
C	3	97.7	68.5
D	2	101.6	60.8
Mean		93.8	59.0

From Levy and Tsuchiya (1972)

Levy and Tsuchiya (1972) also found, however, that aspirin given in *solution* form was very rapidly absorbed into the body as a whole. In such a case, charcoal administration after even 1 or 2 hours would probably have little effect.

Neuvonen, Elfving, and Elonen (1978) have, in fact, shown that when 50g charcoal was given immediately after 1g aspirin to adult subjects, aspirin absorption was decreased 70% relative to control values; yet, when the charcoal was delayed for 1 hour, the reduction in absorption was only 10%. Levy and Tsuchiya also showed conclusively that the presence of food in the digestive tract decreased the effectiveness of activated charcoal. The most likely explanation for this is that the food either provides somewhat of a physical barrier around some of the charcoal, or itself (or breakdown products from it) adsorbs to the charcoal and hence uses up part of the charcoal's capacity.

Collombel and Perrot (1970) carried out studies on sodium salicylate absorption versus delay time in rats. Their results suggest that the charcoal is quite effective at 30 minutes, somewhat effective at 60 minutes, and ineffective at 120 minutes.

Fiser et al. (1971), using studies with dogs, have found that charcoal given after 30 minutes was effective in reducing blood levels of secobarbital, phenobarbital, and glutethimide by an average of 53, 56 and 74%, respectively, over the period of 1–24 hours. They also investigated, for secobarbital only, the effect of waiting 1 hour before giving the charcoal. In this case, the charcoal had very little effect. The reason for this is that secobarbital is relatively quickly absorbed into the body.

Dordoni et al. (1973) found that charcoal, given immediately, reduced the total absorption of acetaminophen into the body by 63%. However, when the charcoal was given I hour after acetaminophen administration, the total uptake into the body was reduced by only 23%. Therefore, with acetaminophen, a delay of even 60 minutes results in much-reduced effectiveness.

TABLE 6:
Effect of Single and Repeated Charcoal Doses on Blood Barbital Concentrations (mg/100 ml)

CHARCOAL TREATMENT	Time periods in hours				
	1	12	24	48	72
None	9.5	8.5	8.0	5.5	4.2
30 minutes	9.1	7.7	7.1	5.5	4.2
1 minute	2.7	4.5	3.5	3.0	2.2
1 minute + 12 hours	3.8	4.9	3.7	2.6	1.6
1 minute, 12 hours, 24 hours	3.4	5.0	3.9	2.2	2.3

Adapted from Chin, Picchioni, and Duplisse (1970)

A similar study with sodium barbital was done with human subjects by Chin, Picchioni, and Duplisse (1970). They studied the effect of delayed and repeated doses on blood barbital concentrations in dogs. The drug dose was 80mg/kg and each charcoal dose was 400mg/kg in suspension. Their results are shown in Table 6. These results clearly show that a time delay of 30 minutes seriously reduces the effectiveness of charcoal, since the barbital is rapidly absorbed. They also show that the additional doses at 12 hours and 24 hours really don't have much, if any, added effect. Perhaps additional doses given earlier (say, at 1 hour, 2 hours, etc.) would have made more of a difference. One study in which repeated doses were given more frequently is that of Andersen (1948c). He gave sulfanilamide to dogs, followed by activated charcoal at intervals of either 15, 45, or 60 minutes. Figure 2 shows blood sul-

fanilamide concentrations versus time. These results show clearly
that charcoal given more frequently has positive benefits, particularly over the first 10 hours.

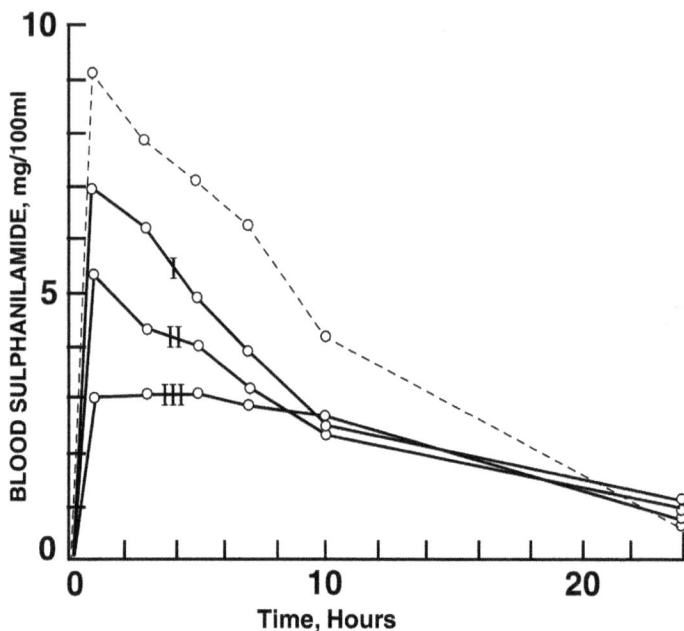

*FIGURE 2. Sulfinilamide concentration in the blood of a dog after
administration of 2g sulfinilamide (upper dashed curve), and the
same amount of sulfanilamide plus 8g charcoal at intervals of 15
(III), 45 (II), and 60 minutes (I). From Andersen, 1948c).*

The fact that various drugs are affected differently by delays
in charcoal administration is shown clearly by the results of Neuvonen, Elfving, and Elonen (1978). When charcoal (50g) was given
immediately after three drugs digoxin (0.5mg), phenytoin (0.5g),
and aspirin (1g)—drug absorption into the body decreased by 98,
98, and 70% respectively, relative to the amounts absorbed when
no charcoal was given. When the charcoal was delayed for 1 hour,
the reductions fell to 40, 80, and 10% respectively. Thus, the delay
had relatively little effect on phenytoin, a drug which is absorbed
slowly by the body. However, for aspirin, which is absorbed fairly

rapidly, the delay has a great effect on the effectiveness of the charcoal.

Drugs which undergo enterohepatic recycling (see Glossary), such as glutethimide, some cardiac glycosides, and tricyclic antidepressants, can be effectively treated by delayed or additional repeated doses of activated charcoal. For example, Belz and Bader (1974) found that the blood levels of intravenously-given methyl proscillaridin (a cardiac glycoside) were effectively and consistently reduced for 48 hours when charcoal was administered three times a day. Similarly, Crome et al. (1977) found that multiple doses of charcoal (at 1/2, 2, 4, and 6 hours) were much more effective in reducing blood levels of the antidepressant nortriptyline than single doses given at 1/2 hour. Figure 3 shows some typical results.

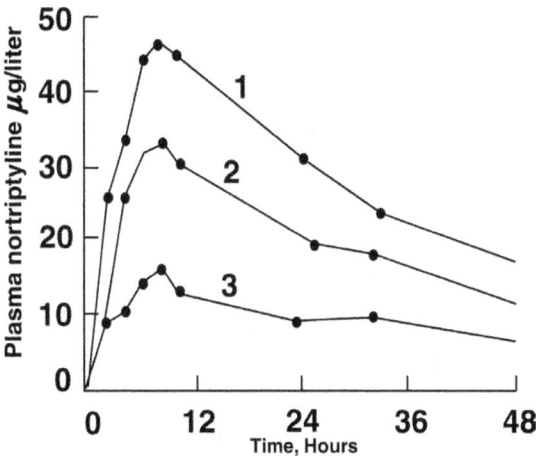

FIGURE 3. Plasma nortriptyline levels after a dose of 75mg nortriptyline in a human subject without charcoal (curve 1), with a single dose of 5g charcoal at 30 minutes (curve 2), and with multiple 5g doses of charcoal at 30, 120, 240 and 360 minutes (curve 3). Adapted from Crome, Dawling, and Braithwaite, 1977.

A year later, Dawling, Crome, and Braithwaite (1978) reported that when 10g of an activated charcoal preparation was given 30 minutes, 2 hours, and 4 hours after giving 75mg nortriptyline to adult subjects, drug uptakes by the body as a whole were decreased by 74, 38, and 13% relative to control values, respectively. Also, peak drug levels in the blood were lowered to 23, 63, and 81% of the control levels. Clearly, the charcoal was quite effective after 30 minutes delay, and much less so for longer delays. However, it is still well worth giving the charcoal even after 4 hours time.

It should be mentioned that many drugs, such as sedatives, hypnotics, and tricyclic antidepressants, tend to reduce gastric contractions and, therefore, the rate of drug absorption. In such cases, charcoal given after some delay can still be of great benefit.

V. STORAGE STABILITY OF CHARCOAL SUSPENSIONS

Although warnings have occasionally been given that a charcoal suspension in water must be prepared immediately before use or else its adsorption ability will be impaired, these have no known basis in fact. The chemical groups (e.g., oxides) which exist on the internal surfaces of activated charcoals have specific affinities for organic chemicals, and the presence of a small unadsorbable substance like water does not destroy this.

To prove this point, Picchioni, Chin, and Laird (1974) tested the strychnine adsorption ability of a freshly prepared charcoal suspension against that of aqueous suspensions that were 3, 6, and 12 months old. The stored suspensions were, if anything, better (8% better on the average, but this difference was not statistically significant).

As long as a suspension is stored in a closed container, so that the adsorption of any substances from air is prevented, the potency of the suspension will be preserved indefinitely.

VI. TOXICITY OF ACTIVATED CHARCOAL

As Hayden and Comstock (1975) have discussed clearly, powdered charcoal has been studied for toxicity due to ingestion, skin contact, and inhalation. All studies show it to be harmless. Nau,

Neal, and Stembridge (1958a) have found that feeding powdered charcoal mixed with dog chow to animals for extended periods of time produced no adverse effects. Nau, Neal, and Stembridge (1958b) have also reported that applications of powdered charcoal to healthy skins of monkeys, mice, and rabbits produced no changes from normal. Nau et al. (1962) similarly found that mice and monkeys exposed by inhalation to powdered charcoal for periods of up to 1900 hours showed no changes in lung tissue; however, emphysema did result simply from the accumulation of the powder in the lung air spaces.

In clinical experiments, Yatzidis and Oreopoulos (1976) relate that kidney disease patients were given 20-50g activated charcoal per day for up to 4 months without any side effects. In fact, it was noted that "the patients had a marked subjective improvement in gastrointestinal symptoms and signs, such as anorexia (appetite loss), nausea, and vomiting. The constipating effect of charcoal was overcome easily by either sorbitol or paraffin oil." In a similar study, Friedman et al. (1978) fed 35g per day of charcoal to six adult patients for up to 2 months and found that "all patients accepted charcoal therapy without difficulty or adverse reaction. There was no apparent interference in appetite, sleep pattern, or general well-being that could be attributed to charcoal ingestion."

Powdered charcoal has been studied for toxicity due to ingestion, skin contact, and inhalation. All studies show it to be harmless.

Chapter 6, Section IX, presents a summary of research which indicates that powdered, activated charcoal has *beneficial* effects on the human gastrointestinal tract.

Wehr et al. (1975) have carefully studied the lung condition of workers in activated charcoal manufacturing plants and found definite radiographic evidence of pneumoconiosis (chronic reaction to dust collection) in 9.6% of the subjects. However, even with extensive bronchial dust accumulation, minimal fibrosis was noted. Also, the incidence of respiratory symptoms in the population was remarkably low, and dust accumulation was not a significant determinant of any pulmonary functional parameter, nor was it an important factor in the production of respiratory tract symptoms. Thus, the authors concluded that even chronic exposure to activated charcoal dust is relatively harmless.

Powdered, activated charcoal has beneficial effects on the human gastrointestinal tract.

It is therefore safe to say that properly manufactured medicinal charcoals seem to pose no hazard. By medicinal charcoals we mean those that have been acid washed so as to extract acid-soluble inorganic materials. This avoids leaching out of these materials, some of which might be harmful, when the charcoal subsequently contacts the gastric fluid in a patient.

Chapter 5
Effects of Activated Charcoal on Various Types of Drugs and Poisons

In this chapter, the discussion of studies on certain specific drugs or classes of drugs is presented. Included will be consideration of common household chemicals, alkaloids, aspirin and other salicylates, hypnotics and sedatives, tricyclic antidepressants, cardiac glycosides, solvents, and a few other specific drugs or poisons such as propoxyphene, ethanol, theophylline, bilirubin, and ethylene glycol.

I. COMMON HOUSEHOLD CHEMICALS

Decker, Combs, and Corby (1968) performed some basic studies in laboratory glassware (as opposed to studies in living persons or animals) on a wide range of poisons, most of which are commonly found in the home. Their experiments involved adding the drugs to 100ml simulated gastric juice, then mixing in 5g Norit A charcoal in 50ml water, and shaking the resultant mixture at

37°C for 20 minutes. The charcoal was separated from the liquid by filtration. Then the clarified liquid was analyzed for residual drug. Drugs supplied in tablet form were crushed beforehand to assure dispersal.

Table 7 shows the percentage of drug absorbed versus the number of tablets used. It was also determined that iodine and phenol (a constituent of calamine lotion) are well adsorbed: chlorpromazine, methyl salicylate, and 2,4 dichlorophenoxyacetic acid are moderately adsorbed; and malathion, DDT, N-methylcarbamate, and boric acid are poorly adsorbed. Mineral acids, alkalis, and compounds insoluble in a water solution (such as tolbutamide) are not adsorbed to any measurable extent.

TABLE 7:
*Drug Adsorption by Activated Charcoal**

| | | Number of Tablets | |
Drug	Dose(mg)	10	20
Acetylsalicylic acid	325	90	85
Amphetamine	5	94	92
Chlorpheniramine	4	96	96
Colchicine	0.5	94	92
Diphenylhydantoin	100	90	86
Ergotamine	1	92	90
Phenobarbital	32	86	45
Primaquine	25	97	94
Propoxyphene	32	100	85
Digitoxin	100	66	60
Probenicid	100	58	40
Quinacrine	325	68	26
Acetaminophen	325	23	8
Glutethimide	500	45	—

| Drug | Dose(mg) | Number of Tablets | |
		10	20
Meprobamate	400	25	—
Propylthiouracil	50	33	23
Qunidine	325	44	1
Quinine	325	32	1
Phenylbutazone	100	15	—
Ferrous Sulfate	325	5	1
Chloroquine	500	6	—

* Values expressed as percent drug adsorbed after 20 minutes. From Corby and Decker (1974); copyright American Academy of Pediatrics, 1974.

Anderson (1946) conducted similar laboratory studies with various drugs and poisons. He determined the maximum amounts that charcoal could adsorb (in milligrams of drug or poison per gram of charcoal). By fitting his Q versus C data to the Langmuir Equation, discussed earlier, he determined values of Q_m (the maximum adsorption capacity of the charcoal) for each chemical. Table 8 shows his results.

TABLE 8:
Maximum Amounts of Substances Adsorbed on Charcoal

Substance	Amount Adsorbed (mg/g)
Mercuric chloride	1,800
Sulfanilamide	1,000
Strychnine nitrate	950
Morphine hydrochloride	800
Atropine sulfate	700

Substance	Amount Adsorbed (mg/g)
Nicotine	700
Barbital	700
Sodium barbital	150
Five other sodium or calcium salts of barbiturates	300-350
Salicylic acid	550
Phenot	400
Alcohol	300
Potassium cyanide	35

From Andersen (1946)

Gloxhuber (1968) has stated that activated charcoal can be used advantageously in cases where detergents and cleansing agents have been ingested.

II. ALKALOIDS

Various alkaloids (mostly strychnine, but also morphine and nicotine) were used in the period of 1920–1940 as standard test substances for the evaluation of medicinal charcoals. As early as 1920, Joachimoglu (1920) showed that charcoal could effectively nullify the effects of strychnine given to dogs. Dingemanse and Lacqueur (1926) did similar studies with pigs, and Kunzova (1937) performed experiments with frogs.

Andersen (1946) used strychnine nitrate, morphine hydrochloride, atropine sulfate, and nicotine in his laboratory glassware studies. Maximum adsorbances for these were 950, 800, 700, and 700mg per gram charcoal, respectively (see Table 8). Other work with alkaloids has been done by Picchioni et al. (1966). They studied strychnine dosed rats. Strychnine phosphate was also given to rats in a similar study by Chin, Picchioni, and Duplisse (1969). These two studies with rats showed that charcoal, in sufficient amounts, was an excellent antidote for strychnine. Henschler

(1970) tested the effectiveness of charcoal in alkaloid poisoning with mice. He found that the ratio of LD_{50} values (see Glossary) with charcoal to LD_{50} values without charcoal were 4.3, 18.2, 3.0, 2.3, 2.5, and 5.5 for six different alkaloids.

III. ASPIRIN AND OTHER SALICYLATES

Decker, Corby, and Ibanez (1968) carried out experiments with rats. When 125mg activated charcoal was administered 30 minutes after a dose of 320mg sodium salicylate, the blood salicylate concentrations at 60, 90, and 120 minutes were reduced by 66, 62, and 62%, respectively, compared to animals which were not given charcoal. Additional work with dogs gave similar results. Figure 4 shows the results of the studies with dogs.

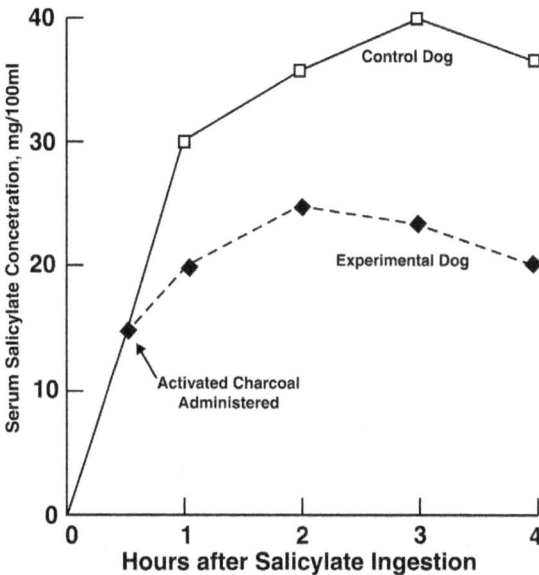

FIGURE 4. Effect of activated charcoal on blood salicylate concentrations in dogs. From Corby, Fiser, and Decker, 1970.

Studies by Decker et al. (1969) in humans also showed a significant inhibition of aspirin absorption. Oral administration of 30g activated charcoal to adult male volunteers 30 minutes after they had received 50 grains of aspirin resulted in blood salicylate concentrations roughly 50% of those in a control group.

Phansalkar and Holt (1968) found that dogs given 100 grains of aspirin plus either 60g or 90g activated charcoal had blood salicylate concentrations that were very small (6–10%) compared to dogs not given charcoal. However, it should be noted that the charcoal-to-drug ratios were roughly 11:1 and 14:1, respectively, so it is not surprising that the reduction in salicylate levels were so large. Even when charcoal was delayed for 1/2 hour, the charcoal abruptly halted the rise in plasma salicylate levels.

Collombel and Perrot (1970) showed in experiments with rats which were given 100mg/kg aspirin that 1g/kg charcoal was capable of lowering blood salicylate levels to varying degrees, depending on the time the charcoal was given. Table 9 clearly shows the effect of the time of charcoal administration.

TABLE 9:
Salicylate Levels (mg/liter) in Rats

Hours since aspirin dose	No Charcoal	Charcoal at 30 min.	Charcoal at 60 min.	Charcoal at 120 min.
1	150	80	160	188
2	240	83	153	230
4	290	85	138	231
8	235	70	103	215
12	140	34	65	103
24	20	15	29	24

From Collombel and Perrot (1970).

Chin, Picchioni, and Duplisse (1969) have reported on studies with dogs. Aspirin, 100mg/kg in an aqueous suspension of 3ml/kg, was administered by stomach tube to four groups of eight dogs each. One minute later three of the groups were treated with activated charcoal (500mg/kg), Arizona montmorillonite (a type of clay), or evaporated milk. Blood samples taken at various times showed that only the activated charcoal was significantly effective in reducing aspirin levels. Chin, Picchioni, and Duplisse (1970) later repeated these experiments with aspirin, as well as with various other drugs. The dosages and the delays in charcoal administration were the same as in their 1969 study, and the results were very similar.

Picchioni, Chin, and Laird (1974) also repeated the aspirin studies in rats. Again the dosages were 100mg/kg aspirin, 500mg/kg charcoal (given after a 1-minute delay). Blood samples taken at 30 minutes showed salicylate levels of 22.3, 8.8, and 4.2mg/100ml for the untreated group and two groups treated with different kinds of charcoal, respectively.

Levy and Tsuchiya (1969, 1972) have reported on studies with aspirin and human subjects. They found that charcoal, if administered promptly and in sufficient amounts, significantly inhibited the absorption of aspirin from a liquid solution, conventional tablets, coated tablets, and sustained release tablets. The effects increased with the amount of charcoal given, decreased as the time delay between the aspirin and charcoal increased, and were decreased by the presence of food in the gastrointestinal tract. Levy and Tsuchiya also showed that charcoal will reduce aspirin absorption even if administered 3 hours after aspirin ingestion, provided that the drug is still in the gastrointestinal tract at that time.

Another study on aspirin is that of Neuvonen, Elfving, and Elonen (1978). Six adults were given 1g aspirin followed by 50g Norit A charcoal. When the charcoal was given immediately, the peak blood aspirin levels were reduced by 95% relative to values for subjects receiving no charcoal.

IV. ACETAMINOPHEN

Acetaminophen is an effective nonprescription, antipyretic, and mild analgesic agent which is being used more and more extensively in the United States. In England (where it is called paracetomol), it has been quite popular for some time, and a history of overdoses has become established. While acetaminophen is very safe in ordinary doses, persons who have ingested large doses (15g or more) develop liver damage. Kidney and heart muscle damage have also been observed. The maximum harmful effect appears 2–4 days after drug ingestion and death can occur between 2 and 7 days after the overdose. Other than the oral administration of either methionine or preferably Nacetylcysteine, two agents which have been found to be specific antidotes for acetaminophen overdoses, only activated charcoal has been shown to be of therapeutic value in preventing liver cell damage or death. Thus, we wish to survey here the limited number of studies done to date which show that activated charcoal may be of great value in counteracting this drug.

The first work in living subjects reported was a brief study by Levy and Gwill (1972) in which it was stated that 10g activated charcoal administered immediately after ingestion of 1g acetaminophen by two human subjects resulted in 77 and 69% reductions in the amounts of drug absorbed from the gastrointestinal tract.

A year later Dordoni et al. (1973) reported on experiments in which 2g oral doses of acetaminophen were given to 14 human subjects. Seven of the subjects were then given 10g activated charcoal as a suspension in methyl cellulose solution (10g/100ml). The charcoal resulted in much lower blood concentrations, and the total uptake of the drug by the body measured as the area under the blood concentration versus time curve over the period 0–120 minutes) was reduced by an average of 63% (range 32–87%). In additional tests, the charcoal was given 60 minutes after acetaminophen ingestion. In these cases, the uptake into the body as a whole (determined for the 60–120 minute period) averaged 23% less for the charcoal treated subjects, as compared to the untreated subjects. The charcoal was, therefore, only about one-third as effective when its administration was delayed an hour.

Another extensive set of results on the in vivo adsorption of acetaminophen in humans is that reported by Levy and Houston (1976). One grain of acetominophen was given to volunteers as an elixir (Tylenol). In one set of experiments 200ml water was then given. In the other experiments each subject was immediately given a slurry of 5 or 10g Norit powdered charcoal in 200ml water. In all tests, urine samples were collected at set times up to 36 hours and were assayed for total acetaminophen (i.e., acetaminophen and its metabolites). The uptakes into the body (determined by the excretion in the urine), relative to those found for the elixir without charcoal, were 52.8 and 38.5% for the 5 and 10g charcoal doses, respectively. Clearly, the charcoal was quite effective.

Levy and Houston (1976) also did a series of tests with humans where the ratio of drug to charcoal was held at 1:10, but different amounts of each were given. Table 10 shows the results. Previous studies by Levy and Tsuchiya (1972) on aspirin showed the same trend shown here, i.e., the effectiveness of charcoal increases with the amount of charcoal even when the ratio of drug to charcoal is held constant.

TABLE 10:

Effect of Charcoal Dose on Acetaminophen at Constant Drug/Charcoal Ratio of 1:10*

Charcoal Dose	Percent acetaminophen absorbed into the body as a whole
5	42.5
10	34.9
20	22.6
30	14.8

*Drug given as elixer followed immediately by charcoal in 200ml water (same sub-jects in all tests). From Levy and Houston (1976); copyright American Academy of Pediatrics, 1976.

Another factor which favors the effectiveness of charcoal in acute acetaminophen overdose is that this drug inhibits gastric emptying, just as aspirin overdoses have been found to do (Levy and Tsuchiya, 1972). This in turn slows down the drug's absorption and suggests that activated charcoal administered even 2–3 hours after the drug ingestion may be significantly effective. Levy and Houston (1976) recommend, based on their results, that a dose of 50–100g activated charcoal should be administered to adults (and proportionately less to children) in acetaminophen overdose cases. Whether reducing the total amount absorbed, or only slowing the rate of absorption of the drug (e.g., lowering the peak blood concentration) would reduce liver damage is not known. It has not yet been shown whether it is the total amount of drug which is harmful or whether it is the peak concentration which is more critical. In either case, the use of activated charcoal would seem to be an effective therapeutic tool.

Other experiments with acetaminophen have been done by Lipscomb and Widdop (1975) using pigs. The acetaminophen (10g) was given either in the form of a liquid suspension or tablets. Half of the pigs were then given 50g activated charcoal in 250ml water. The results of several experiments showed that (1) the drug absorption from the suspension form is much faster than from the tablet form, (2) activated charcoal reduces blood drug concentrations considerably if given at once, and (3) even if delayed for 1/2 or 1 hour, activated charcoal still gives a very significant subsequent reduction in blood levels. One interesting fact that was noted was that, while the pigs' blood levels were often at what would be toxic levels for humans, no evidence of liver damage was noted.

V.   HYPNOTICS AND SEDATIVES

Except for the very early work by Andersen (1947, 1948a), the first studies with hypnotics and sedatives in living subjects were performed by Picchioni's research group. In 1966, they (Picchioni et al., 1966), using rats, studied the adsorption of pentobarbital by one brand of activated charcoal. They later (Picchioni, Chin, and Laird, 1974) did more studies with rats using pentobarbital and three brands of activated charcoals. Another study (Chin et al., 1973) reported on studies in which rats were given barbital and then various amounts of charcoal. Yet another study (Chin,

Picchioni, and Duplisse, 1970) involved experiments using dogs and various drugs, among which were pentobarbital, barbital, and glutethimide. Figure 5 shows one typical set of blood drug concentrations, for barbital. The drug dose was 80mg/kg. The charcoal (given at 1-minute time) amounts were five times the drug amounts. It is clear that the charcoal, at the 5:1 ratio of charcoal to drug, was effective in lowering blood drug levels.

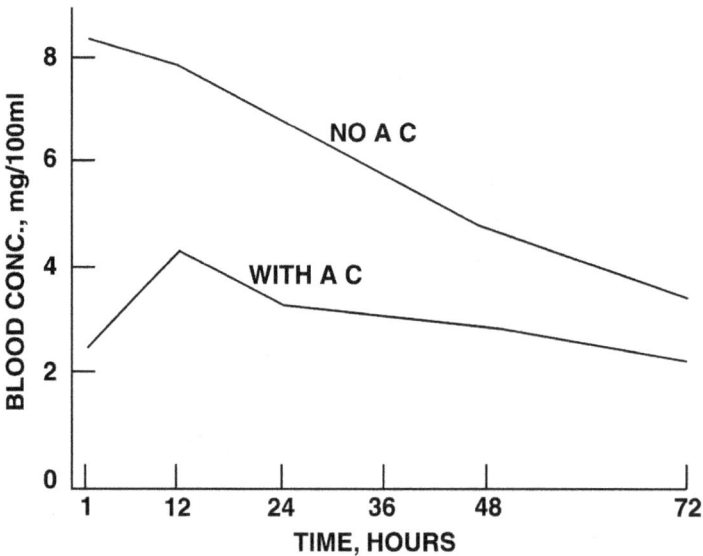

FIGURE 5. *Effect of 5:1 ratio of activated charcoal on blood concentrations of barbital in dogs. Charcoal was given 1 minute after the drug. Adapted from Chin, Picchioni, and Duplisse, 1970.*

A similar study with dogs is that of Fiser et al. (1971) in which doses of secobarbital (400mg), phenobarbital (72mg/kg), or glutethimide (3g) were used. In the first study, no charcoal was given; 2 weeks later the same dogs were given the same drugs plus 20g charcoal 1/2 hour later. The mean reductions in blood drug concentrations over the period 1–24 hours were found to be for secobarbital, 53%; for phenobarbital, 56%; and for glutethimide, 74%. Clearly, charcoal was very effective.

Andersen (1973) gave 40mg/kg diethyl barbituric acid to pigs, then administered 2g/kg activated charcoal. Even when the charcoal was delayed for 8 hours, it "considerably reduced" the absorption of the drug. Also, gastric lavage with a granular suspension in water was effective when carried out within 1 hour, whereas lavage with water alone was without effect.

Lipscomb and Widdop (1975) carried out work in which pigs were given an amobarbital suspension, without charcoal or with charcoal 30 minutes later, and pigs which were given amobarbital capsules, without charcoal or with charcoal 1 hour or 4 hours later. The pigs not receiving the charcoal showed the common clinical response of a lapse into coma, a gradual regaining of consciousness which increased intestinal activity (and therefore speeded up drug absorption), and subsequent relapsing into coma again. The pigs receiving charcoal, even after 4 hours, did not suffer such relapses. Blood drug concentration measurements also confirmed that the charcoal was effective in reducing absorption.

VI. TRICYCLIC ANTIDEPRESSANTS

Crammer and Davies (1972) were perhaps the first investigators to seriously consider the use of activated charcoal in treating overdoses of this class of drugs. They pointed out that the revival of patients poisoned by excessive doses of tricyclic antidepressants is difficult since these drugs are rapidly absorbed from the stomach. Until the normal processes of metabolism and urinary excretion clear the drug (which may take several days), one is faced with having to prevent possible convulsions, dangerously low blood pressure, heart beat irregularities, and so forth.

However, within the body, these drugs undergo enterohepatic circulation (see Glossary). Significant amounts are secreted into the bile, are carried into the upper intestine, and are reabsorbed from the intestines into the blood. It occurred to Crammer and Davies that by use of a suitable adsorbent these drugs might be trapped in the intestines and held there until excretion in the feces.

Rauws and van Noordwijk (1972) have reported on experiments in which rats were given parenteral (non-oral) infusions of imipramine. Certain rats were pretreated with orally administered charcoal; other rats served as the control group. The parenteral route of drug administration was chosen to prevent adsorption of the drug to charcoal prior to intestinal absorption, and thereby indicate if the charcoal could successfully intercept the enterohepatic circulation of the drug. Table 11 shows ratios of the drug concentrations found in various organs of the pretreated rats compared to levels in the same organs of the control rats.

Although these results show some variation, it seems clear that the charcoal was in most cases effective in moderately lowering organ imipramine levels.

TABLE 11:
Imipramine Ratios (Pretreated/Control)

	Intravenous infusion			Intraperitoneal infusion			Mean
	A	B	C	D	E	F	
Heart	0.54	0.90	0.70	0.47	1.00	0.92	0.75
Liver	0.60	0.94	0.85	0.76	1.10	1.10	0.87
Lungs	0.72	0.70	0.75	0.74	0.84	0.66	0.73

From Rauws and van Noordwijk (1972).

A year later, Alvan (1973) described the first reported studies in humans. Six healthy volunteers were given nortriptyline in doses of 0.86–1.00mg/kg on two separate occasions. On one occasion, the drug was followed 30 minutes later with 5g charcoal in a commercially available suspension. Blood samples were taken at 0, 2, 4,12, 24, 32, 48, 56, and 84 hours in both tests. Alvan's results showed reductions due to charcoal in the areas under the blood nortriptyline versus time curves over the span of 0–84 hours of 0, 5, 19, 27, 50, and 72% for the six subjects. Peak blood concentrations were reduced by the charcoal anywhere from about 4 to 69%. While these results are again mixed in nature, it does appear that on average the use of charcoal can significantly reduce nortriptyline levels.

Other very positive results with humans have been reported by Crome et al. (1977). These same results were also reported, in abbreviated form, in a paper by Braithwaite, Crome, and Dawling (1978). They gave 75mg nortriptyline plus a glass of water to healthy volunteers, followed 30 minutes later by 5g activated charcoal contained in a 10g packet of an effervescent charcoal preparation (Medicoal) along with 400 ml more water. In a similar study, multiple charcoal doses of this same size were given at 30, 120, 240, and 360 minutes after drug administration. Typical blood nortriptyline concentrations versus time in untreated and charcoal-treated subjects showed that, for the single charcoal dose study, average reductions in the peak blood drug concentrations were 59%. For the multiple charcoal dose studies, the average peak blood concentration reduction was 72%. In another related study, by Dawling, Crome, and Braithwaite (1978), adults were given 75mg nortriptyline, then a single 10g packet of Medicoal at 30 minutes, 2 hours, or 4 hours. Peak blood concentrations fell by 77, 37, and 19%, respectively. Certainly these results show a substantial favorable effect of charcoal on a representative tricyclic antidepressant in humans.

The extrapolation of Crome's results to doses that are more typical of an overdose (3g or one hundred twenty 25mg tablets at most) represents an uncertainty. However, with an overdose, the effects of these drugs in reducing gastrointestinal contractions may significantly slow down the rate of adsorption. Activated charcoal may be able to reduce adsorption several hours after the overdose has been taken.

Activated charcoal may be able to reduce absorption several hours after the overdose has been taken.

Based on Crome's demonstration that 5g charcoal had a sizable effect in lowering drug levels after a 75mg dose of nortriptyline, it would appear then that for each gram of such a drug taken one should administer 67g charcoal (5 divided by 0.075). This is not an unduly large amount to administer, particularly down a lavage tube to an unconscious patient. It thus appears that activated charcoal can be of significant therapeutic use in tricyclic antidepressant overdoses, if enough is employed.

VII. CARDIAC GLYCOSIDES

For the treatment of severe accidental or suicidal glycoside intoxication, adsorption to activated charcoal has been recommended. Since most cardiac glycosides undergo enterohepatic circulation, adsorbent treatment is suitable not only for oral but also for intravenous glycoside intoxication. For example, Haacke, Johnson, and Kolenda (1973) have estimated that a toxic dose of from 2 to 4mg digitoxin could be satisfactorily counteracted by an oral dose of 30g activated charcoal or 40g cholestyramine (a synthetic resin that can adsorb certain drugs).

In the same year, Härtel, Manninen, and Reissel (1973) reported on a study in which healthy male volunteers were given either 0.5mg digoxin or 0.5mg digoxin plus (5 minutes later) 2g activated charcoal suspended in water. Figure 6 shows the blood digoxin levels measured. It is apparent that the charcoal did significantly reduce the blood digoxin levels. Härtel, Manninen, and Reissell mention that charcoal may be even more effective in digitoxin overdose since this glycoside undergoes substantial enterohepatic circulation (this occurs with digoxin only to a minor degree).

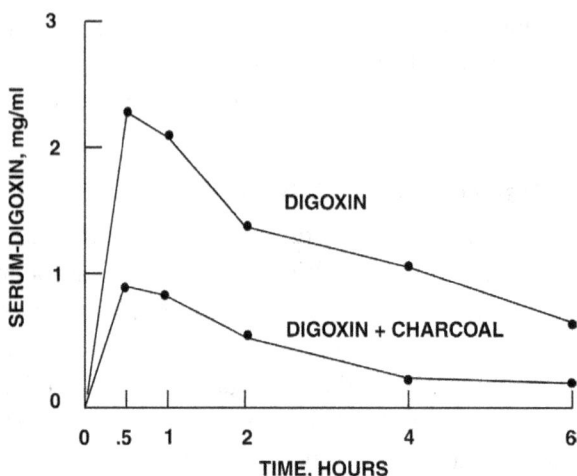

FIGURE 6. *Mean serum levels of digoxin in six healthy subjects after ingestion of 0.5mg digoxin and 0.5mg digoxin plus 2g charcoal. (From Härtel, Manninen, and Reissel, 1973.)*

In 1974, Belz and coworkers reported on three studies involving various glycosides. In one study (Belz and Bader, 1974), healthy volunteers were given 1mg methyl proscillaridin intravenously two times (21 days apart). During one of the periods they received 2g activated charcoal three times per day. Blood glycoside levels over the 48 hours following the drug administration were measured. These data show that on average the drug concentrations were reduced about 40% by charcoal during the period from 10 to 48 hours. Thus, it is clear that methyl proscillaridin undergoes bile excretion and extensive enterohepatic circulation. Therefore, charcoal shows definite promise for treating overdoses of this drug.

More recent work on a cardiac glycoside is the study of Neuvonen, Elfving, and Elonen (1978), in which six adults were given 0.5mg digoxin, followed by 50g Norit A charcoal. When the charcoal was given immediately, the systemic absorption of the digoxin was reduced by 98% relative to patients receiving no charcoal. Even when the charcoal was delayed one hour, a 40% reduction occurred.

VIII. SOLVENTS

Overdoses of solvents such as gasoline, kerosene, lighter fluids, and cleaning fluids are of considerable concern. Especially frequent are cases of children ingesting kerosene in rural or less-developed areas where kerosene is commonly used for cooking, heating and lighting. The most common clinical manifestations of solvent poisoning involve the lungs and central nervous system. Although it is known that solvents are absorbed from the gastrointestinal tract, it is still not clear whether damage to the lungs occurs primarily from the solvent absorbed into the blood or whether primary aspiration, or aspiration secondary to regurgitation, is more important. Various investigators have presented experimental evidence from animal studies favoring either absorption or aspiration as the more damaging process. The consensus seems to be that aspiration is certainly very damaging and that absorption may or may not be of similar importance.

Fortunately, the lethal dose of such solvents seems to be relatively large. Ashkenazi and Berman (1961) state that kerosene poisoning in Israel, though frequent, is rarely fatal. McNally (1956) also offers the view that "it is difficult to conceive of a child drinking a sufficient quantity of kerosene to produce a fatality by absorption from the gastrointestinal tract alone. For a child of 50 pounds a volume in excess of one pint would be the minimal lethal dose without aspiration." Working with rabbits, Diechman et al. (1944) found the lethal dose for this animal to be 28 ml/kg.

Ashkenazi and Berman (1961) have shown that the administration of mineral oil (which remains essentially unabsorbed in the gut) greatly reduced the absorption of kerosene given to rats. However, other reports dealing with various oils (mineral oil, castor oil, olive oil) suggest the opposite. Since our primary concern here is to review studies related to the effects of activated charcoal on solvent poisoning, we shall focus only on charcoal.

One of the best studies reported to date is that of Chin, Picchioni, and Duplisse (1969) in which 8ml/kg (6.4g/kg) kerosene was administered by oral intubation to two groups of 50 rats each.

One minute later one of the groups was treated with 3.6g/kg activated charcoal. As Figure 7 shows, the charcoal was quite effective in reducing blood levels even though the ratio of the weights of charcoal to kerosene was only 0.56.

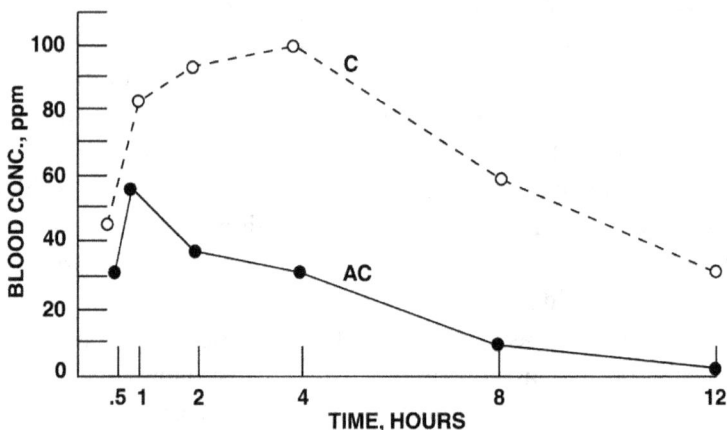

FIGURE 7. *Effect of activated charcoal on blood concentration of kerosene in rats. Key: AC, Charcoal-treated rats; C, control rats. From Chin, Picchioni, and Duplisse, 1969.*

Another study has been described by Laass (1974), who administered lethal doses of various solvents to rats. The doses used were 10ml/kg benzene, tetrachloroethane, or carbon tetrachloride and 5ml/kg diethyl aniline or tetrachloroethane (only one solvent was given to each rat). Following administration of these by oral intubation, each rat was then given either 40ml/kg physiological saline (sodium chloride, NaCl, in water) or 40ml/kg of a suspension of 10% (wt/vol) activated charcoal in water. The lifetimes of the rats are shown in Table 12. Survival times were increased by an average of 166% (range 30–420%) when charcoal was used. Clearly, this is a significant effect. if more charcoal had been given, it is quite likely that some of the rats would have survived.

TABLE 12:
Mean Survival Times in Hours for Rats Given Various Solutions

Solvent	Dose (mg/kg)	+40 ml/kg NaCl	+40ml/kg 10% charcoal
Benzene	10	0.98	2.63
Diethylaniline	10	5.88	10.85
Tetrachloroethane	10	0.15	0.44
Carbon Tetrachloride	10	18.83	38.10
Diethylaniline	5	9.21	11.96
Tetrachloroethane	5	0.14	0.75

Adapted from Laass (1974).

IX. PROPOXYPHENE

Propoxyphene hydrochloride (Darvon, Lilly), a frequently prescribed pain killer, has recently begun to be involved in significant numbers of deaths due to over dosage (e.g., 270 such deaths were reported in 1974 for one population area of 53 million persons). Approximately 20 million prescriptions per year are written for this drug.

Corby and Decker (1968a, 1974) reported that propoxyphene was very well adsorbed from simulated gastric juice by Norit A activated charcoal. They stated that they found 100% adsorption of 10 capsules and 85% adsorption of 20 capsules (each capsule = 32 mg) after 20 minutes in a 150ml solution to which 5g activated charcoal had been added.

Also in 1968, Corby and Decker (1968b) reported that the timely administration of activated charcoal prevented clinical symptoms of propoxyphene poisoning in dogs. The dogs did not have convulsions, nor did they appear to have muscle twitches or respiratory depression.

Chernish, Wolen, and Rodda (1972) have done extensive studies with propoxyphene. Studies were done with six adult men.

They were given 130mg propoxyphene hydrochloride orally with or without 4g activated charcoal. Drug levels in the blood showed that more than half of the drug was prevented from absorbing (Chernish estimates 80mg of the 130mg dose was effectively bound). It appears, then, that charcoal is effective with this drug if enough is used (note that the charcoal/drug ratio was 4:0.13, or 30.7 in this study).

X. BILIRUBIN

Neonatal jaundice caused by excess bilirubin in the blood occurs relatively frequently in premature infants. Its cause is thought to be the inefficient removal of bilirubin by the liver. Several investigators have considered whether orally administered charcoal would be effective in adsorbing bilirubin secreted into the digestive tract (in the bile), thereby preventing its re absorption. Kuenzer, Schenck, and Vahlenkamp (1963) found that charcoal adsorbs bilirubin well from duodenal fluid in laboratory glassware tests. Luecking and Kuenzer (1966) gave charcoal orally to premature infants and found that at a dosage of 1g per day only part of the bilirubin was bound, whereas at a dosage of 4.5g per day bilirubin was so well adsorbed that only a small amount of free bilirubin appeared in the stool. Ulstrom and Eisenklam (1964) have found that if charcoal feeding was started at 12 hours of age, no difference in bilirubinemia (excess bilirubin) occurred between test and control infants. However, when the first dose of charcoal was given at age 4 hours, the charcoal-fed infants had significantly less bilirubinemia than the controls. This suggests that enterohepatic circulation of bilirubin may play a more critical role in determining the amount of bilirubin in the body during the first few hours of life than it does a short time later.

XI. ETHYLENE GLYCOL

Permanent antifreeze and summer coolant is roughly 95% ethylene glycol, and it has been estimated that 40–60 deaths per year result from its accidental or suicidal ingestion. Szabuniewicz,

Bailey, and Wiersig (1975) have reported on a study in which 35 dogs were given 10ml/kg antifreeze. Fifteen were then given 5g/kg activated charcoal, fifteen were treated with ethanol or sodium bicarbonate, and five were left untreated. In these three groups the survivors were 15 of 15, 3 of 15, and 0 of 5, respectively. Clearly, the charcoal was effective. This is somewhat surprising since, as Cooney (1977) has pointed out, ethylene glycol adsorbs poorly to charcoal. He estimated that only 3.6% of the ethylene glycol would be bound by the charcoal. The explanation of charcoal's great effect may be related more to its metabolites, particularly oxalic acid, which may adsorb much better to charcoal. Some type of circulation of the metabolites back into the digestive tract would be required, of course, for contact with the charcoal to occur. Further studies are obviously needed.

XII. ETHANOL

North, Thompson, and Peterson (1981) gave 6 healthy dogs an oral dose of 2ml/kg of ethanol (the alcohol of found in beer, wine, and liquor) in a water solution. Blood ethanol concentrations were then measured at 0.5, 1, 2, 3, and 6 hours. A week later the tests were repeated (same dogs), only 50g of activated charcoal in water was given just prior to the ethanol dose. The results showed that activated charcoal greatly reduced ethanol absorption into the body as a whole, especially during the first 2 hours. Since ethanol is a simple chemical and would not be expected to adsorb well to charcoal, these results are difficult to explain. Therefore, it appears that additional research will be needed to clarify the mechanism whereby the charcoal slurry had the observed effect.

XIII. THEOPHYLLINE

Theophylline produces bronchodilation and is widely used to treat diseases of reversible airway obstruction (e.g., asthma). Because of the ready availability and increased usage of this drug, plus the fact that there is a narrow range between beneficial amounts and harmful amounts, frequent acute overdoses can be expected, especially among children. For these reasons, Sintek, Hendeles, and Weinberger (1978,1979) have studied theophylline adsorption by activated charcoal. These investigators gave adult men and women 500–600mg of theophylline plus 30g activated charcoal in slurry form 30 minutes later. Absorption "then appeared to stop abruptly." By comparison to control tests (no charcoal given) it was found that the charcoal decreased theophylline absorption by an average of 59%. However, the decreases ranged from 26 to 96% for the 5 subjects, probably because of a great variability in the amount of drug absorbed in the 30 minutes prior to the charcoal administration. On balance it is clear that the dose of charcoal delivered (30 g) was quite effective, even after a delay of 30 minutes.

XIV. OTHER DRUGS OR POISONS

Other drugs or poisons which have been studied with respect to them in vitro or in vivo adsorption to activated charcoal and which do not fall within any of the previous classifications are listed in Table 13. We shall not discuss these here, and merely cite them for the sake of completeness.

TABLE 13:
Other Drugs or Poisons Studied

Investigators	Drug or Poison	In vitro/ vivo
De Souza et al. (1973)	Chlorpheniramine maleate	In vitro
Picchioni, Chin, and Laird (1974)	Chlorpheniramine maleate	In vivo
Chin, Picchioni, and Duplisse (1970)	Chlorpheniramine maleate, chloroquine, chlorpromazine	In vivo
Tsuchiya and Levy	Phenylpropanolamine, salicylamide	In vitro/ vivo

Investigators	Drug or Poison	In vitro/ vivo
Otto and Stenberg (1973)	Salicylamide	In vitro/ vivo
Ivan (1972)	Sulfanilamides	In vitro
Andersen (1948a)	Sulfanilamides	In vivo
Andersen (1948b)	Allylpropynol	In vivo
Atkinson and Azarnoff	Neguvon	In vivo
Picchioni et al. (1966)	Malathion	In vitro/ vivo
Smith et al. (1967)	D-amphetamine, tripelennamine, ferrous sulfate, ethanol	In vitro
Chin et al. (1973)	Chloroquine, isonazid	In vivo
Edwards and McCredie (1967)	Meprobamate carbromal, bromine, iodine	In vitro
Sellars, Khouw, and Dorman (1977)	Chlordiazepoxide, diazepam, methaqualone	In vitro
Sorby (1961, 1965, 1966)	Phenothiazine derivatives	In vitro
Boehm, Brown, and Oppenheim (1978)	Pheniramine maleate	In vivo
Boehm and Oppenheim (1977)	Pheniramine maleate, thioridazine hydrochloride	In vitro
Sandvordeker and Dajani (1975)	Diphenoxylate hydrochloride	In vitro/ vivo
Chaput de Saintonge and Herxheimer	Propantheline	In vivo
Picchioni and Consroe (1979)	Phencyclidine	In vivo
Neuvonen, Elfving, and Elonen	Diphenylhydantoin	In vivo
Ganjian, Cutie, and Jochsberger (1980)	Cimetidine	In vitro

Chapter 6
Other Medicinal Uses of Charcoal

Activated charcoal has a long history of medical applications other than as an oral antidote. For example, it has been shown that activated charcoal can adsorb bacteria, viruses, bacterial toxins, snake venoms, and various other biochemicals. Charcoal has also shown beneficial action in the treatment of skin wounds.

Activated charcoal can adsorb bacteria, viruses, bacterial toxins, snake venoms, and various other biochemicals.

Surprisingly, most of the applications just mentioned were developed and studied in the period from about 1910 to the late 1930s. From 1940 onward, references to such applications are very few in number. However, it is entirely possible that some of the concepts proposed so long ago might have application today. For the purpose of bringing this older work to the attention of present-day audiences, we shall now review some of the studies in the various areas of application mentioned above.

I.   SNAKE VENOM ADSORPTION

Houssay (1921) was apparently the first person to report on the adsorption of snake venom components by charcoal. She found, in laboratory studies, that the hemolytic substance (i.e., one that destroys red blood cells) of snake venoms is adsorbed by charcoal.

Boquet (1928) also studied the adsorption of cobra venom by charcoal. Fifty milligrams of desiccated cobra venom was dissolved in 50ml physiological salt solution, and 1g of sterilized activated charcoal was added and mixed in well. After 2 hours the suspension was filtered, and the suspension and the filtrate were found to be equally harmless. Injections equivalent to 100 fatal doses had no venomous action. This inactivation of venom by charcoal was independent of temperature between 12 and 38°C, and required only 8–10 seconds of contact. Neither heat to 70°C for 30 minutes nor acids, 0.2–0.5ml of 0.1 N HCI per 10 ml, liberated the venom bound to the charcoal. Tests with diphtheria toxin gave similar results.

Thrash and Thrash (1981) recommend charcoal poultices as well as oral charcoal for snakebites and state that they know of physicians who have used it successfully. However, they give no specific details of the physicians' experiences.

II.   VIRUS ADSORPTION

Poppe and Busch (1930) showed that three strains of foot-and-mouth disease viruses were capable of adsorbing to charcoal so strongly that none of the supernatants (the relatively clear fluids which exist above the charcoal after the charcoal is allowed to settle) were infectious upon injection into guinea pigs.

Cordier (1939) later reported that foot-and-mouth disease virus in a 1% suspension of the virus in a physiological solution can be entirely adsorbed on charcoal if the charcoal is used in the amount of 10g charcoal per l00ml fluid. The virus is not destroyed, but its activity is much reduced. Injections of the virus-charcoal complex were found to create immunity to the virus. Cordier (1940) further indicates that sheep pox virus is also adsorbed by charcoal. This has been confirmed by Stamatin (1937) who earlier also studied sheep pox virus adsorption on charcoal.

III. BACTERIA ADSORPTION

Wiechowski (1914) was one of the first to report that "charcoal is capable, not only in the test tube but in the human body, of adsorbing...bacteria...thereby preventing...their poisonous action." Salus (1916) wrote of experiments in which contaminated water was shaken with charcoal and then filtered through paper. The filtrate was generally free of bacteria, although when milk or blood was used as the fluid, such was not the case. He also observed that *cocci* were better adsorbed than typhoid bacteria and the latter better than *Bacillus coli.*

Oksent'yan (1940) reported that up to 90–100% of *Thermobacterium halveticum, Streptococcus lactis,* and *Saccaromyces ellipsoideus* are adsorbed by various charcoals. Adsorption was not found to affect the reproduction of the bacteria, but it did sharply lower their physiological functions.

Gunnison and Marshall (1937) found that charcoal could remove *L. acidophilus* and *staphylococci*, but not *E. coli* or *C. welchii,* from suspension. Gram-positive organisms did not generally adsorb any better than gram-negative ones. It was concluded that clinical improvements observed following the administration of adsorbents are probably due to the adsorption of bacterial toxins or enzymes rather than the bacterial cells themselves.

IV. BACTERIAL TOXIN ADSORPTION

Kraus and Barbera (1915) have demonstrated the excellent binding of diphtheria toxin to charcoal by contacting a 10% solution of the toxin with the charcoal for 1 hour, and then injecting the supernate subcutaneously into a guinea pig. The animal survived without even showing local swelling, whereas a control animal died within 48 hours from 1% as much toxin. Similar results were obtained with tetanus and dysentery. A study of the same nature on diphtheria toxin by Boquet (1928) has already been mentioned above in the discussion of snake venom adsorption. Signorelli (1933) has reported that charcoal is capable of diminishing the toxic properties of tuberculin toxin, as well as of tetanus toxin.

Siebert (1935) found that a purified tuberculin protein derivative was not itself able to stimulate antibody production. However, when injected in particulate form after adsorption to charcoal, it became truly antigenic (i.e., stimulated antibody production).

Hemolysins for sheep red blood cells were found to quantitatively adsorb from rabbit serum to charcoal, according to a study by Roffo and Barbera (1925).

More recently, Drucker et al. (1977) have discussed very clearcut evidence that activated charcoal prevents the toxic effects of endotoxins produced by *Vibrio cholera* and *Escherica coli.* When the adsorbents and isolated toxins were either preincubated together or injected simultaneously into the intestinal loops of rabbits, no toxic effects occurred. However, when the whole bacterial cells were used, rather than the isolated toxins, toxic reactions did occur in most cases.

V. FUNGUS TOXIN ADSORPTION

Aflatoxin B_1 Toxin is a deadly toxin produced by the fungus *Aspergillus flavus* which is commonly found growing as mold on corn, peanuts, and seeds such as cottonseed. Animals, and occasionally humans, have died as a result of eating such contaminated plants. Decker and Corby (1980) have shown that activated charcoal can adsorb aflatoxin efficiently in vitro. Hatch et al. (1982) have shown that lethal doses (3mg/kg) given to goats could be counteracted completely (zero deaths) by immediate administration of a charcoal slurry. it seems likely that humans could also be treated effectively by prompt oral charcoal use.

Mushroom poisoning, due to a toxin produced by the deadly mushroom *Amanita phalloides,* can be effectively counteracted by hemoperfusion (see Section XI) over granular activated charcoal, as shown by Wauters, Rossel, and Farquet (1978). No research using orally administered powdered charcoal has been reported to date, but these hemoperfusion results strongly suggest that oral charcoal would also be effective in mushroom poisoning, if given early enough.

VI. CHARCOAL FOR TREATING SURFACE WOUNDS AND INSECT BITES/STINGS

In addition to the reference to Kehls (1793) mentioned under Section II in Chapter 2, in which the external application of charcoal to gangrenous ulcers for removal of bad odors was cited, several other works suggesting the use of charcoal for treating surface wounds have appeared. Schobesch (1938) indicates that aqueous solutions or pastes of yperite (dichlorodiethyl sulfide) readily irritated the skin of rabbits. Activated charcoal, applied to such injured areas, was the most effective treatment found. Even after a 10-minute delay, good results were obtained. Peyer (1940) has reported that "coffee chars" are effective on various surface wounds. however, Riedel (1940) has suggested that the therapeutic value of charcoals derived from coffee could not be due to their adsorptive powers, since he found that they were not very large. However, he does agree that the coffee charcoals are for some reason therapeutic.

The most scientific study carried out on the effect of activated charcoal in treating wounds is one reported by Beckett et al. (1980). They used an activated charcoal cloth (made by pyrolizing a rayon fabric and then activating the resulting charred cloth by exposure to an oxidizing agent). Twenty-six patients with chronic leg ulcers and 13 patients with suppurating post-operative wounds had the charcoal cloth applied as a dressing. All wounds initially were infected, were discharging fluid, and were malodorous. Wound odor was reduced noticeably in 95% of the patients, and self-cleansing of the wounds occurred in 80% of the patients. No adverse reactions to the charcoal occurred; nor did the cloth adhere to the wounds and cause any difficulties in removal of the dressing. In vitro experiments with patches of the cloth dropped into solutions of bacteria showed that bacterial counts in the solutions decreased by 1000– to 100,000-fold due to binding of the bacteria by the cloth. Hence, it appears that bacterial adsorption by the cloth accounts for its effectiveness as a wound dressing.

Thrash and Thrash (1981) give various recipes for charcoal poultices. A basic poultice can be prepared by adding 1 tablespoon ground flaxseed and 1 tablespoon charcoal powder into 1/3 cup of water, mixing thoroughly, letting the mixture set for 10–20 minutes, and heating it slightly to thicken. The mixture is then spread 1/4-inch thick between two layers of cloth (leaving a clear area near the edges). After placing the cloth patch on the affected area, it should be covered with plastic wrap, and then covered with a roller bandage to hold it in place. It should be left on for 6–10 hours. For larger areas, the recipe can be doubled or tripled. For very small areas, the recipe can be cut back or, as an alternative, a simple paste of only charcoal powder and water can be used.

Bites and stings from ants, spiders, bees, wasps, etc., can be treated effectively using the poultices described above, according to Thrash and Thrash (1981). They state also that the swelling and pain from such bites and stings will be alleviated in roughly 5 minutes. However, especially venomous bites such as from the brown recluse spider will require extended treatment with charcoal poultices.

> *Bites and stings from ants, spiders, bees, wasps, etc., can be treated effectively using the poultices.*

VII. CHARCOAL USE FOR ITCHING

Relief of generalized itching (pruritus) by oral activated charcoal has been reported by Pederson et al. (1980). Eleven artificial kidney patients, who were experiencing pruritus as a side effect of their kidney disease, were given 6g per day activated charcoal by mouth for 8 weeks. The pruritis was relieved in all but one patient. Additionally, scratch-induced skin sores were greatly cleared up. A possible explanation of the charcoal's effect is that it adsorbs compounds producing the pruritis, in the gastrointestinal tract. No adverse effects of the charcoal were noted; hence, it is highly recommended for relieving itching conditions.

VIII. REDISCOVERY OF THE EFFECT OF ACTIVATED CHARCOAL UPON ABDOMINAL INFECTIONS

Whereas the ability of activated charcoal to adsorb bacterial toxins was well-known and fairly extensively studied in the period from 1910 to the mid-1930s, its value in treating infections of the digestive tract seems since then to have been unappreciated, if not forgotten. It is therefore very interesting to note that in 1978 a paper by Kopp appeared having the title "The unexpected success of enteral activated carbon in acute renal failure patients in the prevention and therapy of abdominal sepsis."

Kopp states that the sequence of paralysis of the ileum (lower small intestine), toxic inflammation of the peritoneum (membrane lining the abdominal cavity), and endotoxin shock, has been one of the major unconquered and frustrating problems in the treatment of patients with acute kidney failure. Despite heroic attempts, these complications invariably have led to death. The use of charcoal in treating drug intoxications gave Kopp the idea of trying it for toxic abdominal infection. He states:

The results are indeed impressive. Toxic degradation products within the intestinal lumen [inner channel] are efficiently adsorbed. Paralytic small and large bowel distension disappears, toxic damage to the liver and...the "spill over" phenomenon of bacterial toxins into the systemic circulation are obviously prevented. Other conventional attempts, e.g., whole gut sterilization, etc., were non successful in our experience. Survival of patients has been achieved in a number of cases even in the presence of incipient abdominal catastrophe, using enteral [intraintestinal] carbon. The results have also important implications in the management of surgical and trauma patients in general.

IX. CHARCOAL FOR INTESTINAL DISORDERS

Some impressive evidence that activated charcoal can be effective in treating various intestinal disorders has recently been reported by Chervil (1978). Using a mixture called Carbomucil-30g activated charcoal powder, 14g magnesium bicarbonate, 33g sterculia gum, and 100g excipient—Chevrel studied its effects, when given a minimum of twice per day, on a variety of intestinal disorders, such as diarrhea, constipation, cramps, and flatulence. In 60 cases, excellent results (all troubles gone in 2–4 weeks) were achieved in 70% of them and very good results (notable amelioration, but requiring more than 4 weeks treatment) were obtained in another 15%. Only 15% of the cases showed little or no improvement. While the Carbomucil ingredients other than the charcoal might have been of real importance, there are substantial reasons for believing that the activated charcoal was the crucial substance. Certainly, further studies of this type with varied formulations seem warranted.

Hall, Thompson, and Strother (1981) gave 13 human adult subjects various types of meals, with or without activated charcoal, over a period of several weeks. The meals were: (1) a "normal" meal, (2) a high gas-producing bean meal followed by 3 capsules of activated charcoal (194mg in each capsule) immediately plus 3 more capsules after 2 hours, (3) a high gas-producing bean meal followed by 3 starch-filled placebo capsules immediately plus 3 more placebo capsules after 2 hours. The study was done in a double-blind manner. Breath hydrogen was measured periodically in all subjects (hydrogen is produced in the body almost entirely by bacterial action in the GI tract, from where it is absorbed in the blood and carried to the lungs for excretion in the breath). Over the period from 0–7 hours, the mean number of "flatus events" resulting from the three meals cited above were 3.0, 2.7, and 14.5 respectively. Breath hydrogen levels were elevated after 4 hours' time in the "bean meal plus placebo" case, and were essentially the same for the other two meals. It was concluded that the use of activated charcoal can keep gas production at normal levels even when a high gas-producing type of meal is consumed.

Sebedo et al. (1982) studied the effect of activated charcoal (Norit) on diarrhea in 39 children in Indonesia. Group 1 (23 children) received only oral glucose electrolyte solution (this combats the severe dehydration resulting from diarrhea). Group 11 (16 children) received the oral glucose solution plus a dose of the activated charcoal (166mg to 750 mg, depending on body weight, 3 times/day). The charcoal lowered the duration of diarrhea from 3.0 days to 2.1 days, a reduction of 30%. It may be that a much larger activated charcoal dose would have had a bigger effect. Unfortunately, only fairly low charcoal doses were employed.

X. CHARCOAL FOR OSTOMY IMPROVEMENT

Kappeler et al. (1984) tested the effect of an activated charcoal preparation [15g activated charcoal plus 12g sorbitol sweetener and some excipient (inert material to provide thicker consistency) in 100ml water] on stool consistency, flatulence, and odor in 93 patients with intestinal stomas (an opening created surgically in the abdominal wall through which intestinal matter is excreted, rather than having it pass through the lower intestines and rectum). More than two-thirds of the patients had improved stool consistency, reduced flatulence, and reduced odor. A granular charcoal preparation (granular charcoal plus bentonite clay) was also tried. Patients with colostomies (in which the opening is connected to the colon, or large intestine) had good results, as before, but patients with ileostomies (in which the opening is connected to the ileum, or small intestine) did not show significant improvement.

Johnson (1977) also mentions the use of activated charcoal capsules three times daily to reduce stool odor and flatulence in patients having colostomies.

XI. HEMOPERFUSION APPLICATIONS

Hemoperfusion is a relatively new medical subject area in which activated charcoals are widely used to treat victims of poisoning or drug overdose. Figure 8 shows the major features of a hemoperfusion circuit. It should be emphasized here that only granular charcoals can be used for hemoperfusion. This fact differentiates this topic from all of the other applications of charcoal mentioned thus far in this book, since all of the other uses involve powdered charcoals. It should also be pointed out that hemoperfusion is complementary to orally administered charcoal powder as a treatment for poisonings or drug overdoses. Powdered charcoal is mainly effective if used while the toxin is still in the stomach. Once absorption into the body as a whole occurs, hemoperfusion may then be the treatment of choice. Thus, powdered charcoal is useful at "early times" and hemoperfusion at "later times."

Powdered charcoal is mainly effective if used while the toxin is still in the stomach.

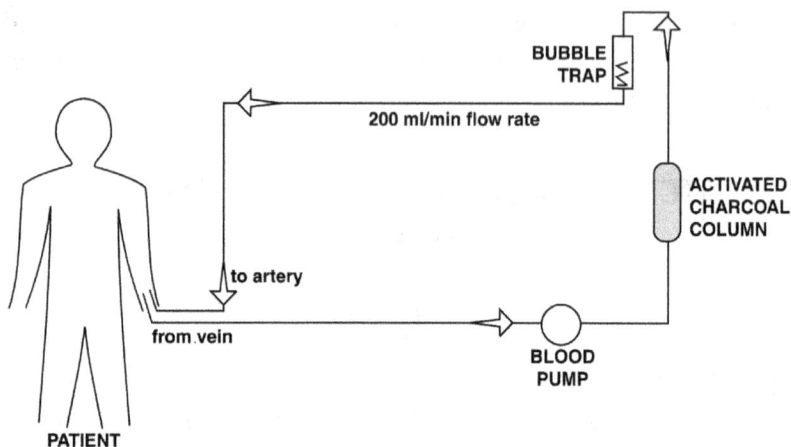

FIGURE 8. Typical hemoperfusion system

The published literature relating to hemoperfusion is by now quite extensive. Approximately 400 papers could be cited which deal directly with the subject. Thus, any complete discussion of hemoperfusion would require a publication of a size comparable to the present one. Here, we will only be able to familiarize the reader with the basic nature of hemoperfusion and its main applications.

The concept of flowing blood over activated charcoal granules to remove unwanted substances seems to have originated with Yatzidis (1964), who used a column of 200g of 0.50–0.75 mm diameter granules to hemoperfuse dogs at a blood-flow rate of 50–100 ml/min for up to 90 minutes duration. It was found that creatinine, uric acid, phenolic compounds, guanidine bases, and organic acids were all removed well. Yatzidis mentioned the possible use of such a system in removing endogenous toxins (those produced *inside* the body, as in kidney or liver failure), as well as exogenous toxins (those arising from *outside* the body, such as drugs or poisons). Work by Andrade et al. (1971, 1972) showed that, even with very extensive preliminary washing of a charcoal bed, fine particles are released, due to the rubbing together of the charcoal granules. These fine particles are dangerous in that they can plug up small blood vessels in the body. Several investigators suggested using various polymer coatings to prevent fine carbon particle release. Chang et al. (1969) suggested using nylon, collodion, or heparin-complexed collodion; Denti, Luboz, and Tessore (1975) proposed cellulose acetate; and Andrade (1971, 1972) tested an acrylic hydrogel and albumin cross-linked with glutaraldehyde. All of these coatings were successful in preventing fine particle release; moreover, some of the coatings were "bio-compatible" enough with blood so that blood cell damage during hemoperfusion was decreased to tolerable levels.

Within the last few years, a few hemoperfusion columns have been developed to the point where they are now commercially marketed. Some of the drugs which have been found to be effectively removed by some or all of the hemoperfusion devices are barbiturates, glutethimide, methyprylon, meprobamate, ethchlorvynol, acetaminophen, salicylates, chloral hydrate, digitalis, mipramineI, nortriptyline, meproscillaridin, and diazepam. In addition, various poisons have been effectively removed by hemoperfusion, including organophosphates, paraquat, (an herbicide), paralytic shellfish poisons, insecticides, carbon tetrachloride, and mushroom toxins. Endogenous species removed well by hemoperfusion include (1) excess thyroid hormones in cases of "thyroid storm"; (2) various uremic (kidney disease) metabolites such as creatinine and uric acid (3) various species which accumulate during liver failure, such as bilirubin, bile acids, and certain amino acids and (4) bacterial toxins. Excess amounts of methotrexate, an anticancer agent, have also been removed by charcoal hemoperfusion. As a general rule, it would appear that any chemical that has been found to be well adsorbed by powdered charcoal would also be adsorbed well in a granular charcoal hemoperfusion column.

XII. PROLONGATION OF LIFESPAN

Frolkis et al. (1984) recently reported some extremely interesting results on the effect of oral charcoal on prolonging the life span of "old" (28-month-old) rats. Since toxic metabolites are believed to play a role in aging, the purification of digestive juices in the intestinal tract using activated charcoal ("enterosorption") could potentially remove such toxic substances from a person's system.

Different amounts of activated charcoal in the rats' diets, increased the rats' mean life spans at 50%, 80%, and 100%

Enterosorption, using different amounts of activated charcoal in the rats' diets, increased the rats' mean life spans at 50%, 80%, and 100% mortality by 47%, 41%, and 44%, respectively, as compared to controls. It increased their maximal life spans by 34%, as compared to controls.

The charcoal also decreased the rate' of onset of age-related structural and metabolic changes, e.g. heart myofibrosis was less marked, sclerosis of the renal glomeruli was absent, and similar age-related changes in the liver, pancreas, and lungs were either absent or much less than those found in the control animals. Decreases in blood cholesterol and triglycerides were found in the treated animals (as has been seen in humans). RNARNA and protein biosynthesis in the liver was found to increase.

Further research is needed to determine if the dramatic effect of enteric activated charcoal is due to the adsorption of known or supposed metabolites, or due to changes in the amounts of physiologically active substances and subsequent regulatory transformations, or both.

Chapter 7
Summary

There can be no doubt that activated charcoal as an antidote is generally very effective in preventing the systemic absorption of a wide variety of drugs and poisons.

We have pointed out certain guidelines for its use: a medicinal grade (acid-washed), powdered, activated charcoal should be selected, and it should be given as soon as possible in amounts that are as large as the person will accept (100g minimum, if possible). The charcoal should be made more easily ingested

There can be no doubt that activated charcoal as an antidote is generally very effective in preventing the systemic absorption of a wide variety of drugs and poisons.

by being mixed with sufficient amounts of water. While charcoal ingestion can cause some minor constipation to occur in the intestinal tract, this problem can be easily counteracted by appropriate doses of laxative agents such as mineral oils.

Our review of the uses of activated charcoal from 1500 B.C. to the present reveals the rather surprising fact that the merits of activated charcoal have often not been fully appreciated. This is especially true of the period from about 1930 to the present. This has led to a continuous cycle of the rediscovery and disappearance of its use. Hopefully, the current new cycle of awareness of activated charcoal's powers will soon result in (1) there being a container of antidotal charcoal in every home and emergency room, and (2) there being a return to (and further research on) the use of activated charcoal for promoting the general health of the gastrointestinal tract.

REFERENCES

Alvan, G. (1973). Effect of activated charcoal on plasma levels of nortriptyline after single doses in man. *Eur. J. Clin. Pharmacol.* 5:236.

Andersen, A. H. (1946). The pharmacology of activated charcoal. I. Adsorption power of charcoal in aqueous solutions. *Acta Pharmacol. Toxicol.* 2:69.

Andersen, A. H. (1947). The pharmacology of activated charcoal. II. Effect of pH on adsorption by charcoal from aqueous solutions. *Acta Pharmacol. Toxicol.* 3:199.

Andersen, A. H. (1948a). Pharmacology of activated charcoal. III. Adsorption in presence of gastrointestinal contents. *Acta Pharmacol. Toxicol.* 4:275.

Andersen, A. H. (1948b). Pharmacology of activated charcoal. IV. Adsorption of allylisopropylbarbituric acid in vivo. *Acta Pharmacol. Toxicol.* 4:379.

Andersen, A. H. (1948c). Pharmacology of activated charcoal. V. Adsorption of sulphanilamide in vivo. Acta *Pharmacol. Toxicol.* 4:389.

Andersen, A. H. (1973). Medicinal charcoal in the treatment of poisoning. Treatment of experimental poisoning in pigs. *Ugeskr. Laeger* 135:797.

Andrade, J. D.; Kunitomo, K.; Van Wagenen, R.; Kastiger, B.; Gough, D.; and Kolff, W. J. (1971). Coated adsorbents for direct blood perfusion: HEMA/activated carbon. *Trans. Amer. Soc. Artif. Intern. Organs 17:22.*

Andrade, J. D.; Van Wagenen, R.; Chen, C.; Ghavamian, M.; Voider, J.; Kirkham, R.; and Kolff, W. J. (1972). Coated adsorbents for direct blood perfusion II. *Trans. Amer. Soc. Artif. Intern. Organs* 18:473.

Ashkenazi, A., and Berman, S. E. (1961). Experimental kerosene poisoning in rats, *Pediatrics* 28:642.

Atkinson, J. P., and Azarnoff, D. L. (1971). Comparison of charcoal and attapulgite as gastrointestinal sequestrants in acute drug ingestions. *Clin. Toxicol.* 4:31.

Beckett, R.; Coombs, T. J.; Frost, M. R.; McLeish, J.; and Thompson, K. (1980). Charcoal cloth and malodorous wounds. *Lancet,* September 13, 594.

Belz, G. G., and Bader, H. (1974). Effect of oral charcoal on plasma levels of intravenous methyl proscillaridin. Klin. *Wochenschr.* 52:1134.

Boehm, J. J., and Oppenheim, R. C. (1977). An in vitro study of the adsorption of various drugs by activated charcoal. *Aust. J. Pharm. Sci.* 6:107.

Boehm, J. J.; Brown, T. C. K.; and Oppenheim, R. C. (1978). Reduction of pheniramine toxicity using activated charcoal. *Clin. Toxicol.* 12:523.

Boquet, A. (1928). Adsorption of cobra venom and diphtheria toxin by carbon. *Compt. Rend.* 187:959.

Braithwaite, R. A.; Crome, P.; and Dawling, S. (1978). The in vitro and in vivo evaluation of activated charcoal as an adsorbent for tricyclic antidepressants. *Br. J. Clin. Pharmacol.* 5:369.

Chang, T.M.S.; Gonda, A.; Dirks, J. H.; and Malave, N. (1969). Removal of endogenous and exogenous toxins by a micro encapsulated adsorbent. *Can. J. Physiol. Pharmacol.* 47:1043.

Chaput de Saintonge, D. M., and Herxheimer, A. (1971). Activated charcoal impairs propantheline absorption. *Eur. J. Clin. Pharmacol.* 4:52.

Cheldelin, V. H., and Williams, R. J. (1942). Adsorption of organic compounds. 1. Adsorption of ampholytes on an activated charcoal. *J. Amer. Chem. Soc.* 64:1513.

Chernish, S. M.; Wolen, R. L.; and Rodda, B. E. (1972). Adsorption of propoxyphene hydrochloride by activated charcoal. *Clin. Toxicol.* 5:317.

Chevrel, B. (1978). Traitment des troubles functionnels intestinaux par le carbomucil. *Med. et Chir. Digest(Paris)* 7:443.

Chin, L.; Picchioni, A. L.; and Duplisse, B. R. (1969). Comparative antidotal effectiveness of activated charcoal, Arizona montmorillonite, and evaporated milk. *J. Pharm. Sci.* 58:1353.

Chin, L.; Picchioni, A. L.; and Duplisse, B. R. (1970). Action of activated charcoal on poisons in the digestive tract. *Toxicol. Appl. Pharmacol.* 16:786.

Chin, L.; Picchioni, A. L.; Bourn, W. M.; and Laird, H. E. (1973). Optimal antidotal dose of activated charcoal. *Toxicol. Appl. Pharmacoi.* 26:103.

Collombel, C., and Perrot, L. (1970). Treatment of salicylate poisoning with activated charcoal. *J. Eur. Toxicol.* 3:352.

Comstock, E. (1975). Guide to management of drug overdose. *Clin. Toxicol.* 8:475.

Cooney, D. O. (1977). The treatment of ethylene glycol poisoning with activated charcoal. *IRCS Med. Sci.* 5:265.

Cooney, D. O. (1978). In vitro evidence for ipecac inactivation by activated charcoal. *J. Pharm. Sci.* 67:426.

Cooney, D. O. (1980). *Activated charcoal: Antidotal and Other Medical Uses,* Marcel Dekker, N.Y.

Corby, D. G., and Decker, W. J. (1968a). An antidote for propoxyphene hydrochloride. *JAMA* 203:1074.

Corby, D. G., and Decker, W. J. (1968b). Treatment of propoxyphene poisoning. *JAMA* 205:250.

Corby, D. G., and Decker, W. J. (1974). Management of acute poisoning with activated charcoal. *Pediatrics* 54:324.

Corby, D. G.; Decker, W. J.; Moran, M. J.; and Payne, C. E. (1968). Clinical comparison of pharmacologic emetics in children. *Pediatrics* 42:361.

Corby, D. G.; Fiser, R. H.; and Decker, W. J. (1970). Reevaluation of the use of activated charcoal in the treatment of acute poisoning. *Ped. Clin. N. Amer.* 17:545.

Cordier, G. (1939). Adsorption of the virus of foot and mouth disease by bone carbon and tricalcium phosphate. Applications to the immunization of the cavy. *Red. Med. Vet.* 115:599.

Cordier, G. (1940). Symbiosis "in vivo" of the virus of sheep pox and of the virus of foot and mouth disease. Simultaneous adsorption of the two viruses by animal carbon. *Rec. Med.* Vet. 116:254.

Crammer, J., and Davies, B. (1972). Activated charcoal in tricyclic drug overdoses. *Br. Med. J.* 3:527.

Crome, P.; Dawling, S.; Braithwaite, R. A.; Masters, J.; and Walkey, R. (1977). Effect of activated charcoal on absorption of nortriptyline. *Lancet 2:1203.*

Dawling, S.; Crome, P.; and Braithwaite, R. (1978). Effect of delayed administration of activated charcoal on nortriptyline absorption. *Clin. Pharmacol.* 14:445.

Decker, W. J.; Combs, H. G.; and Corby, D. G. (1968). Adsorption of drugs and poisons by activated charcoal. *Toxicol. Appl. Pharmacol.* 13:454.

Decker, W. J.; Corby, D. G.; and Ibanez, J. D., Jr. (1968). Aspirin adsorption with activated charcoal. *Lancet* 1:754.

Decker, W. J., and Corby, D. G. (1980). Activated charcoal adsorbs aflatoxin B_1. *Vet. Hum. Toxicol.* 22:388.

Decker, W. J.; Shpall, R. A.; Corby, D. G.; Combs, H. F.; and Payne, C. E. (1969). Inhibition of aspirin absorption by activated charcoal and apomorphine. *Clin. Pharmacol. Ther. 10:710.*

Deichman, W. B.; Kitzmuth, K. V.; Witherup, S.; and Joaansmann, K. (1944). Kerosene intoxication. *Arch. Intern. Med.* 21:803.

Deitz, V. R. (1944). Bibliography of Solid Adsorbents, U.S. Cane Sugar Refiners and Bone Char Manufacturers and the National Bureau of Standards, Washington, D.C.

Denti, E.; Luboz, M. P.; and Tessore, V. (1975). Adsorption characteristics of cellulose acetate coated charcoals. *Biomed, Mater. Res.* 9:143.

De Souza, J. J. V.; Mitra, A. K.; Gupta, S.; and Gupta, B. K. (1973). Adsorption of chlorpheniramine maleate from aqueous solution by activated charcoal. *Indian J. Pharm.* 35:167.

Dingemanse, E., and Lacqueur, E. (1926). Adsorption of poisons on charcoal. 111. The distribution of poisons between stomach and intestine wall and charcoal. *Biochem. Z.* 169:235.

Dordoni, B.; Willson, R. A.; Thompson, R. P. H.; and Williams, R. (1973). Reduction of absorption of paracetomol by activated charcoal and cholestyramine: A possible therapeutic measure. *Br. Med. J.* 3:86.

Drucker, M. M.; Goldhar, J.; Ogra, P. L.; and Neter, E. (1977). The effect of attapulgite and charcoal on enterotoxicity of Vibrio cholera and Escherichia coli enterotoxins in rabbits. *Infection 5:211.*

Edwards, D. G., and McCredie, M. (1967). Binding properties of acidic, basic, and neutral drugs to anion and cation exchange resins and charcoal in vitro. *Med. J. Aust.* 1:534.

Fiser, R. H.; Maetz, H. M.; Treuting, J. J.; and Decker, W. J. (1971). Activated charcoal in barbiturate and glutethimide poisoning of the dog. *J. Pediatrics* 78:1045.

Friedman, E. A.; Feinstein, E. I.; Beyer, M. M.; Galonsky, R. S.; and Hirsch, S. R. (1978). Charcoal-induced lipid reduction in uremia. *Kidney Int.* 13 (Suppl. 8), S-170.

Frolkis, V. V. et al. (1984). Enterosorption in prolonging old animal life span. *Exp. Gerontol.* 19:217.

Ganjian, F.; Cutie, A. J.; and Jochsberger, T. (1980). In vitro adsorption studies of cimetidine. *J. Pharm. Sci.* 69:352.

Garrod, A. B. (1846). On purified animal charcoal as an antidote to all vegetable and some mineral poisons. *Trans. Med. Soc. London* 1:195.

Gloxhuber, C. (1968). Treatment after intake of detergents and cleansing agents. *Med. Welt.* 6:351.

Gunnison, J. P., and Marshall, M. S. (1937). Adsorption of bacteria by inert particulate reagents. *J. Bacteriol. 33:401.*

Haacke, H.; Johnson, K.; and Kolenda, K. D. (1973). Therapy of digitalis poisoning: Another experimental indication of the efficiency of adsorbents. *Med. Welt.* 24:1374.

Hall, R. G., Jr.; Thompson, E.; and Strother, A. (1981). Effects of orally administered activated charcoal on intestinal gas. *Am. J. Gastroenterol.* 75:192.

Härtel, G.; Manninen, V.; and Reissell, P. (1973). Treatment of digoxin intoxication. *Lancet* 2:158.

Hassler, J. W. (1963). *Activated Carbon,* Chemical Publishing Co., New York.

Hatch, R. C.; Clark, J. D.; Jain, A. V.; and Weiss, R. (1982). induced acute aflatoxicosis in goats: Treatment with activated charcoal or dual combinations of oxytetracycline, stanozolol, and activated charcoal. *Am. J. Vet. Res.* 43:644.

Hayden, J. W. and Comstock, E. G. (1975). Use of activated charcoal in acute poisoning. *Clin. Toxicol.* 8:515.

Henderson, M. L.; Picchioni, A. L.; and Chin, L. (1966). Evaluation of oral dilution as a first aid measure in poisoning. *J. Pharm. Sci.* 55:1311.

Henschler, D. (1970). Antidotal properties of activated charcoal. *Arh. Hig. Rada Toksikol.* 21:129.

Holt, L. E., Jr., and Holz, P. H. (1963). The black bottle—a consideration of the role of charcoal in the treatment of poisoning in children. *J. Pediatrics* 63:306.

Houssay, M. A. (1921). Adsorption of snake venom by charcoal. *Rev. Inst. Bacteriol. Dep. Nac. Hig. (Buenos Aires)* 2:197.

Ivan, J. (1972). Adsorption of sulphanilamides on activated carbon. *Acta Pharm. Hung.* 42:97.

Joachimoglu, G. (1920). The theoretical principles of charcoal therapy. *Chem.-Ztg.* 44:780.

Johnson, J. B. (1977). Try activated charcoal for ostomates? (letter). *Patient Care,* October 30, p.152.

Kappeler, M.; Rufenacht, R.; Müller, S.; and Halter, F. (1984). [Effect of a charcoal preparation on fecal consistency and odor of patients with intestinal stomas]. *Schweiz. Rundschau Med.* 73:351.

Kehls, D. M. (1793). Memoire sur le charbon vègètal, observations et journal sur la physique, de chemie et I'histoire naturelle et des arts, Paris. *Tome XLII,* 250.

Kopp, K. F. (1978). The unexpected success of enteral activated carbon in acute renal failure patients in the prevention and therapy of abdominal sepsis. *Abstr. Amer. Soc. Artif. Intern. Organs* 7:31.

Kraus, R., and Barbera, B. (1915). Adsorption of toxins by animal charcoal. *Deut. Med. Wochschr.* 41:393.

Kuenzer, W.; Schenck, W.; and Vahlenkamp, H. (1963). Bilirubin adsorption from duodenal fluid by charcoal. *Klin. Wochschr.* 41:1108.

Kunzova, H. (1937). The evaluation and the use of animal charcoals. *Prakticky Lekar 17:337.*

Laass, W. (1974). Suitability of using activated charcoal for the treatment of acute oral poisoning with organic solvents. *Pharmazie* 29:728.

Lawrence, F. H., and McGrew, W. R. (1975). Activated charcoal: A forgotten antidote. *J. Maine Med. Assoc.* 66:311.

Levy, G., and Gwilt, P. (1972). Activated charcoal for acute acetaminophen intoxication. *JAMA* 219:621.

Levy, G., and Houston. J. B. (1976). Effect of activated charcoal on acetaminophen absorption. *Pediatrics* 58:432.

Levy, G.,and Tsuchiya,T. (1969). Effect of activated charcoal on aspirin absorption in man. *Pharmacologist 11:292.*

Levy, G., and Tsuchiya, T. (1972). Effect of activated charcoal on aspirin absorption in man. *Clin. Pharmacol. Ther.* 13:317.

Lipscomb, D. J., and Widdop, B. (1975). Activated charcoal in the treatment of drug overdoses using the pig as an animal model. *Arch. Toxicol.* 34:37.

Luecking, T., and Kuenzer, W. (1966). Absorption of intestinal bilirubin by carbon. *Klin. Wochschr.* 44:469.

McNally, W. D. (1956). Kerosene poisoning in children: A study of 204 cases. *J. Pediatrics* 48:296.

Nau, C. A.; Neal, J.; and Stembridge, V. (1958a). A study of the physiological effects of carbon black. I. Ingestion. *Arch. Ind. Health 17:21.*

Nau, C. A.; Neal, J.; and Stembridge, V. (1958b). A study of the physiological effects of carbon black. II. Skin contact. *Arch. Ind. Health* 18:511.

Nau, C. A.; Neal, J.; Stembridge, V.; and Cooley, R. N. (1962). Physiological effects of carbon black. IV. Inhalation. *Arch. Environ. Health* 4:415.

Neuvonen, P. G.; Elfving, S. M.; and Elonen, E. (1978). Reduction of absorption of digoxin, phenytoin, and aspirin by activated charcoal in man. *Eur. J. Clin. Pharmacol.* 13:213.

North, D. S.; Thompson, J. D.; and Peterson, C. D. (1981). Effect of activated charcoal on ethanol blood levels in dogs. *Am. J. Hosp. Pharm.* 38:864.

Oksent'yan, U. G. (1940). Activity of lactic acid bacteria in connection with adsorption. *Microbiology (USSR)* 9 (No. 1): 3.

Otto, U., and Stenberg, B. (1973). Drug adsorption properties of different activated charcoal dosage forms in vitro and in man. *Sv. Farm. Tidskr.* 77:613.

Pederson, J. A.; Matter, B. J.; Czerwinski, A. W.; and Llach, F. (1980). Relief of idiopathic generalized pruritis in dialysis patients treated with oral activated charcoal. *Ann. Intern. Med.* 93:446.

Peyer, W. (1940). Coffee char and its possibilities. *Pharm: Zentralhalle* 81:1.

Phansalkar, S. V., and Holt, L. E., Jr. (1968). Observations on the immediate treatment of poisoning. *J. Pediatrics* 72:683.

Picchioni, A. L.; Chin, L.; Verhulst, H. L.; and Dieterle, B. (1966). Activated charcoal versus "universal antidote" as an antidote for poisons. *Toxicol. Appl. Pharmacol.* 8:447.

Picchioni, A. L.; Chin, L.; and Laird, H. E. (1974). Activated charcoal preparations: Relative antidotal efficacy. *Clin. Toxicol.* 7:97.

Picchioni, A. L., and Consroe, P. F. (1979). Activated charcoal—a phencyclidine antidote, or hog in dogs. *New Eng. J. Med.* 300(4):202.

Poppe, K., and Busch, G. (1930). Physical and chemical studies of the virus of foot and mouth disease. *Z. Immunitats.* 68:510.

Rand, B. H. (1848). On animal charcoal as an antidote. *Med. Examiner* 4:528.

Rauws, A. G., and Van Noordwijk, J. (1972). Activated charcoal in tricyclic drug overdoses. *Br. Med. J.* 4:298.

Riedel, H. (1940). The adsorptive capacity of coffee carbon. *Klin. Wochschr.* 19:1064.

Robertson, W. O. (1962). Syrup of ipecac: A fast or slow emetic? *Amer. J. Dis. Child* 103:136.

Roffo, A. H., and Barbera, B. (1925) . The adsorption of hemolysins. *Biol. Inst. Med. Exptl. Estud. Cancer 1:280.*

Salus, G. (1916). Blood charcoal as a disinfectant of small quantities of water. *Wien. Klin. Wochschr.* 29:846.

Sandvordeker, D. R., and Dajani, E. Z. (1975). In vitro adsorption of diphenoxylate hydrochloride on activated charcoal and its relation to pharmacological effects of drug in vivo. *J. Pharm. Sci.* 64:1877.

Saunders, F.; Lackner, J. E.; and Schochet, S. S. (1931). Studies in adsorption. I. The adsorption of physiologically active substances by activated charcoal. *J. Pharma*col. 42:169.

Schobesch, O. (1938). Prophylactic treatment of yperite injuries. *Antigaz (Bucharest)* 12:436.

Sears, Roebuck and Co. (1969). 1908 Catalog No. 117 (reprint), Digest Books, Northfield, Illinois, p. 790.

Sebodo, T., et al. (1982). Carbo-adsorbent (Norit) in the treatment of children with diarrhoea, *S. E. Asian J. Trop. Med. Pub. Hlth.* 13, 424.

Sellers, E. M.; Khouw, V., and Dolman, L. (1977). Comparative drug adsorption by activated charcoal. *J. Pharm. Sci.* 66:1640.

Siebert, F. B. (1935). The chemical composition of the active principle of tuberculin: XIX. Difference in the antigenic properties of various tuberculin fractions; adsorption to aluminum hydroxide and charcoal. *J. Immunol.* 28:425.

Signorelli, S. (1933). Adsorption power of carbon on complex toxins and tuberculosis of miners. *Bull. Soc. Ital. Biol. Sper.* 8:116.

Sintek, C.; Hendeles, L.; and Weinberger, M. (1978). Activated charcoal adsorption of theophylline in vitro. *Drug Intell. Clin. Pharm.* 12:158.

Sintek, C.; Hendeles, L.; and Weinberger, M. (1979). inhibition of theophylline absorption by activated charcoal. *J. Pediatrics* 94:314.

Smith, R. P.; Gosselin, R. E., Henderson, J. A.; and Anderson, D. M. (1967). Comparison of the adsorptive properties of activated charcoal and Alaskan montmorillonite for some common poisons. *Toxicol. Appl. Pharmacol.* 10:95.

Sorby, D. L. (1965). Effect of adsorbents on drug absorption: I. Modification of promazine absorption by activated attapulgite and activated charcoal. *J. Pharm. Sci.* 54:677.

Sorby, D. L., and Plein, E. M. (1961). Adsorption of phenothiazine derivatives by kaolin, talc, and Norit. *J. Pharm. Sci.* 50:355.

Sorby, D. L.; Plein, E. M.; and Benmaman, J. D. (1966). Adsorption of phenothiazine derivatives by solid adsorbents. *J. Pharm. Sci.* 55:785.

Stamatin, N. (1937). Adsorption of the sheep-pox virus on kaolin and animal charcoal. *Compt. Rend. Soc. Biol.* 124:984.

Szabuniewicz, M.; Bailey, E. M.; and Wiersig, D. O. (1975). New regimen for the treatment of ethylene glycol poisoning. *IRCS Med. Sci. (Libr. Compend.)* 3:102.

Thrash, A., and Thrash, C. (1981). *Home Remedies,* Chapter 15, "Charcoal Therapy," Thrash Publ., Seale, AL.

Tsuchiya, T., and Levy, G. (1972a). Drug adsorption efficacy of commercial activated charcoal tablets in vitro and in vivo. *J. Pharm. Sci.* 61:624.

Tsuchiya, T., and Levy, G. (1972b). Relation between effect of activated charcoal on drug absorption in man and its drug adsorption characteristics in vitro. *J. Pharm. Sci.* 61:586.

Ulstrom, R. A., and Eisenklam, E. (1964). The enterohepatic shunting of bilirubin in the newborn infant: I. Use of oral activated charcoal to reduce normal serum bilirubin values. *J. Pediatrics 65:27.*

United States Pharmacopoeia, 19th rev. (1975). Mack Printing Co., Easton, PA.

Wauters, J. P.; Rossel, C.; and Farquet, J. J. (1978). Amanita phalloides poisoning treated by early charcoal haemoperfusion. *Br. Med. J.* 2, November 25,1465.

Wehr, K. L.; Johanson, W. G., Jr.; Chapman, J. S.; and Pierce, A. K. (1975). Pneumoconiosis among activated carbon workers. *Arch. Environ. Health* 30:578.

Wiechowski, W. (1914). Pharmacological basis for a therapeutic use of charcoal. *Z. Kinderheilk. 8:285.*

Yatzidis, H. (1964). A convenient haemoperfusion micro apparatus over charcoal for the treatment of endogenous and exogenous intoxication. *Proc. Eur. Dialysis Transpl.* Assoc. 1:83.

Yatzidis, H., and Oreopoulos, D. (1976). Early clinical trials with sorbents. *Kidney Int.* 10 (Suppl. 7):S-215.

GLOSSARY

absorption—the uptake of a chemical (e.g., drug or poison) from the interior of the gastrointestinal tract into the rest of the body, by transfer through the walls of the gastrointestinal tract, passage into the tiny blood vessels on the other side, and subsequent distribution of the chemical to other body regions by the flowing blood.

adsorption—the binding of a chemical (e.g., drug, poison, biochemical, etc.) to a solid material such as activated charcoal, a clay, or a solid synthetic polymeric resin.

alkaloid—one of a large group of bitter-tasting chemicals found in plants. They are usually physiologically active (e.g., caffeine, morphine, strychnine).

analgesic—an agent that alleviates pain without causing loss of consciousness.

antidepressant—an agent that relieves or prevents depression.

antipyretic—an agent that relieves or reduces fever.

aqueous—watery, e.g. pertaining to a solution prepared with water as the main ingredient.

cardiac glycoside—one of a class of chemicals, derived from plants, which have a specific action on the heart (e.g., stimulate the heart).

control—a test or test subject against which experimental observations may be evaluated, identical in all respects to the experimental test or test subject except for the absence of the one factor (e.g., activated charcoal dose) that is being studied.

endogenous—arising from within the body.

enterohepatic recycling—recycling of a chemical by absorption from the intestinal tract into the systemic circulation, followed by extraction of the chemical from the blood by the liver and excretion of the substance into the bile, which then is secreted into the intestinal tract, thereby completing the cycle.

et al.—abbreviation for et alia, Latin for "and others." Used in references to publications to refer to a series of authors following the main author.

exogenous—arising from outside of the body.

g—abbreviation for gram (453.6g = 1 lb).

gastric—pertaining to the stomach.

gastrointestinal tract—the stomach and intestines.

hypnotic—an agent that induces sleep.

inorganic—chemicals derived mainly from mineral matter, usually containing atoms of metallic species.

in vitro—within glassware (i.e., observable in a test tube or similar glass vessel).

in vivo—within a living body (animal, human).

kg—abbreviation for kilogram (1 kg = 1000g = 2.205 lb).

LD_{50}—abbreviation for median lethal dose; a dose which is lethal for 50% of the test subjects.

mesh—particle size expressed in terms of the mesh size of a screen that it will just barely pass through (e.g., a 100 mesh screen has 100 wires per inch horizontally and vertically).

metabolites—chemical substances produced by the metabolic breakdown of a primary substance.

mg—abbreviation for milligram (1/1000th of a gram).

mg/kg—drug or poison dose given to a test subject expressed as milligrams of drug or poison per kilogram of body weight.

ml—abbreviation for milliliter (1/1000th of a liter).

organic—chemicals consisting mainly of carbon, hydrogen, and oxygen atoms, frequently derived from living or formerly-living organisms.

parenteral—delivered by non-oral means (e.g., intramuscularly, intravenously, subcutaneously).

plasma—the fluid portion that remains when blood cells are removed from blood (e.g., by centrifugation).

salicylates—any simple derivative of salicylic acid (e.g., sodium salicylate). Salicylates have analgesic/antipyretic properties.

sedative—an agent that reduces excitement, agitation, and hyper-activity.

serum—the clear liquid that remains when the blood cells and fibrinogen (a protein involved in clotting) have been removed from blood.

slurry—a suspension of a solid powder (e.g., activated charcoal) in a liquid (e.g., water).

systemic—pertaining to the body as a whole.

toxin—a high molecular weight poison produced by some plants, animals, and bacteria which can be inactivated by specific antigens.

wt/vol—concentration of a chemical in a solution expressed as the weight of chemical per unit volume of solution.

Index

We invite you to view the complete
selection of titles we publish at:

www.TEACHServices.com

scan with your mobile
device to go directly
to our website

Please write or email us your praises, reactions, or
thoughts about this or any other book we publish at:

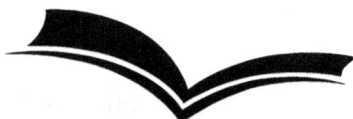

TEACH Services, Inc.
P U B L I S H I N G
www.TEACHServices.com • (800) 367-1844

Info@TEACHServices.com

TEACH Services, Inc., titles may be purchased in bulk for
educational, business, fund-raising, or sales promotional use.
For information, please e-mail:

BulkSales@TEACHServices.com

Finally if you are interested in seeing
your own book in print, please contact us at

publishing@TEACHServices.com

We would be happy to review your manuscript for free.

www.ingramcontent.com/pod-product-compliance
Lightning Source LLC
Chambersburg PA
CBHW072207270326
41930CB00011B/2568